Bring juice or water to a boil. Add salt and chopped fruit. Return to boil and simmer 5 minutes until softened.

COMPOTE 3
Yield: 2½ cups

> ½ **cup prunes**
> ½ **cup raisins**
> 1 **cup water**
> ¼ **tsp sea salt**
> 1 **orange, peeled, seeded, and chopped**

Soak prunes and raisins in water for 15 minutes. Add salt, cover, and bring to a boil. Simmer over low heat for 15 to 20 minutes until plump. Remove form heat and add orange pieces.

RICE SYRUP SAUCE
Yield: 1½ cup

> ½ **cup rice syrup**
> ½ **cup water**
> **pinch sea salt**
> ¼ **tsp cinnamon**
> **approximately 1 Tbsp arrowroot powder diluted**
> **in ¼ cup water**

Boil rice syrup with water, salt, and cinnamon for 2 to 3 minutes. Add diluted arrowroot powder and stir until thickened. Serve.

For additional breakfast recipes, see:
Basic Congee Recipe—Barb Jurecki-Humphrey, page 89.
Morning Cereal and Rice Cream—Ginat Rice, page 103.
Steamed Amaranth and Sarrasin Crepes—Rebecca Wood, page 119.

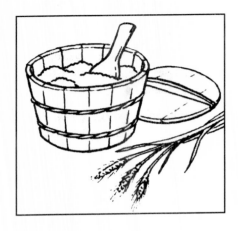

Grain Salads
for Summer

Hot weather and hot stoves don't mix. When the temperatures rises, it is hard to stand by a stove and prepare food, any food actually, and especially foods that require lengthy cooking—grains and beans. Grains and beans are the cornerstone of macrobiotic meals, and, for many people, a day without grains and beans is like a day without sunshine. For this reason, grains and beans are often incorporated into salads at the hot time of year. Salads are refreshing and light; plus, the inclusion of greens, yellows, and oranges adds pleasant colors to grains dishes, lightening them in appearance as well as in flavor.

Grain salads can be made with raw vegetables such as cucumbers, celery, and lettuce or cooked vegetables such as corn, peas, or carrots. When using cooked foods, cool before mixing to avoid excess heat that can spoil a salad.

Serve salads at a comfortable room temperature, or slightly chilled if in a hot climate. It may be tempting to think of consuming cold or chilled foods to balance summer heat yet it is important to use discretion. Chilled and cooled foods taken in excess can weaken the stomach and intestines, dampening digestive fire needed for optimal absorption, and setting the body up for too much internal coolness once autumn arrives.

Rather than "adding cold," think of "reducing heat." In practical terms, this means cooking early in the day before it gets hot and reducing how often you bake. This idea also applies to limiting foods such as animal foods, heavy grain or bean casseroles, hearty vegetable stews, or "too hot" spices that create excess internal heat. Cinnamon and ginger are warming spices that increase internal heat and are best limited in summer. Garlic, cumin, and chili peppers are warming spices that disperse internal heat and can be used on occasion or liberally, as desired. Other herbs and spices can be used to enhance food—both for flavor and for temperature. Dill, basil, cilantro, and other herbs and spices add lightness and freshness.

Grain salads are served at noon-time meals at camp and feature the following recipes. The 5-taste rice uses cooked vegetables. The brown rice salad uses raw. The quinoa salad incorporates red lentils in the salad; the buckwheat salad uses sauerkraut. Tabouli is a classic recipe involving no cooking. Try them all and make variations as desired.

5-TASTE RICE

Yield: 8 cups

Cornellia Aihara served this masterpiece of a brown rice dish often—each year at summer camp and for festivals and potlucks at Vega Study Center. She varied it with the season such as adding cooked burdock or arame in cooler months. It was always colorful and flavorful. She sometimes referred to it as "chirashi-sushi," "5-taste rice," "5-color rice," or "gomaku rice."

Cornellia studied flower arrangement when growing up in Japan and approached meal preparation with similar poise and perfection. She emphasized the importance of serving an odd number of dishes on a plate for a pleasing balance, using 5 or 7 choices—never 4 or 6. She did the same with this dish, aiming to incorporate an odd number of ingredients. Tastes and colors were important too and she would rattle off a list of colors: white rice, black shiso, orange carrot, green scallions, and brown sesame seed. Substitutions were okay as long they coordinated such as black seaweed instead of shiso.

Tastes needed to be varied too. In this dish, soy sauce provides a salty flavor, rice and carrots a sweet flavor, ginger a hot flavor, scallions a pungent flavor, and shiso a sour flavor. While it isn't mandatory to have all 5 tastes every time, she advised me to prepare this dish with at least 3 of the flavors.

This dish continues to be prepared at camp in honor of Cornellia. The preparation is somewhat involved yet well worth the effort.

> **2 cups short grain brown rice**
> **4 cups water**
> **pinch of sea salt**
> **3 to 5 dried shiitake mushrooms, will hydrate to ½ cup**
> **½ cup water**
> **1 teaspoon soy sauce**
> **½ cup roasted sesame seeds or gomashio**
> **1 large carrot, thin quarter rounds**
> **2 cups water**
> **pinch of sea salt**
> **4 Tbsp pickled ginger, minced**
> **2 Tbsp packaged dried shiso powder; or 4 Tbsp dried shiso**
>   **leaf from shiso packed with umeboshi plums, finely**
>   **minced; or 6 Tbsp fresh shiso leaf, finely minced**
> **½ cup finely cut scallion or parsley**

Soak 2 cups brown rice in 4 cups water and 3 to 5 shiitake mushrooms in ½ cup water for 4 to 8 hours.

To cook rice: add sea salt to rice, cover pan, and bring to a boil over medium heat. Simmer 1 hour over low heat using a heat diffuser. Remove from heat and cool. Alternately, if desired, use a pressure cooker to prepare rice. Use 3 cups of water, rather than 4. Pressure cook for 45 minutes following directions as per pressure cooker instructions.

To cook shiitake mushrooms: remove soaked mushrooms from water and reserve water. Remove hard stems and discard (or retain for soup stock), and slice caps into thin crescents. Return to soaking water with the soy sauce, bring to a boil and simmer 15 minutes or until soft. Let water cook away. Cool.

Roast sesame seeds in a dry skillet, 7 to 10 minutes until toasted, stirring frequently. Grind in suribachi or blender until most seeds are crushed.

To cook carrots: bring the 2 cups of water to a boil. Add a small pinch of sea salt and the cut carrots. Return to a boil, then remove and drain. Cool. (Water can be saved for sup stock.)

To assemble 5-taste rice: mix 6 cups cooked, cooled rice with ½ cup cooked shiitake mushrooms, ½ cup roasted sesame seeds or gomashio, 1 cup blanched carrot, 4 tablespoons minced pickled ginger, 2 to 6 tablespoons shiso, and ½ cup finely cut scallion or parsley. Taste, adjust seasonings, adding more shiso, pickled ginger, or parsley, and serve.

Brown Rice Salad
Yield: 4 cups

This is an easy recipe to prepare and lends well to substitutions or additions. Use other cooked grains such as millet or quinoa, add other ingredients such as cooked corn or peas, or garnish with colorful and nutritious adornments such as avocado, tomato, or crumbled nori.

At camp, chickpeas are often served alongside this salad rather than incorporated. Either way is satisfying as the protein in the chickpeas combines with the carbohydrates in the rice to provide complete nutrition.

> ¼ **red onion, finely minced, ¼ cup**
> 1 **Tbsp umeboshi vinegar**
> 3 **Tbsp olive oil**
> 1 **celery stalk, finely diced, ¾ cup**
> ½ **carrot, grated, ¼ cup**
> 3 **cups cooked brown rice, or 2½ cups cooked brown rice and ½**
>   **cup cooked drained garbanzo beans**

Mix red onion and umeboshi vinegar and let sit 10 minutes. Mix in olive oil, celery and carrot. Add cooked brown rice or rice and beans. Let sit 20 minutes before serving. For variation, add chopped olives, minced parsley, sliced radishes, or chopped cucumber. Serve on lettuce leaves.

Quinoa Red Lentil Salad
Yield: 5½ to 6 cups

This salad combines grains and beans for complete nutrition. Cumin and garlic add more flavor; use higher quantities if preferred.

> 3 **cups water**
> ½ **cup red lentils, rinsed and drained**

> 1 cup quinoa, rinsed and drained
> 2 cloves garlic, minced, 1 Tbsp
> ½ tsp ground cumin
> 1 tsp dill weed
> ¼ tsp sea salt
> ½ small red onion, minced, ½ cup
> 1 Tbsp umeboshi vinegar
> 3 Tbsp olive oil
> 1 large celery stalks, minced, ½ cup
> 1 carrot, grated, 1 cup
> 1 Tbsp parsley, finely cut
> ½ cup walnuts, roasted and chopped, optional

Bring 3 cups water to a boil in medium size saucepan. Add lentils, return to a boil with lid ajar on pan. Simmer 5 minutes.

Add quinoa, garlic, cumin, dill weed, and sea salt and simmer 30 minutes until all liquid is absorbed.

Mince red onion and mix with umeboshi vinegar. Let stand for 10 to 15 minutes. Add olive oil, mined celery, and grated carrots to red onion and let marinate while quinoa finishes cooking and cooling. Roast walnuts in skillet for 5 to 6 minutes until fragrant. Cool and chop.

When quinoa has cooled, mix with vegetables, parsley, and walnuts if used. Serve.

BUCKWHEAT SALAD
Yield: 5 to 5½ cups

David and Cynthia Briscoe (*www.macroamerica.com*) presented this recipe at a camp cooking class a number of years ago and received a very favorable review. Buckwheat is a "dry" grain and this salad is especially helpful in hot, humid climates and to decrease water retention.

> 3 cups cooked buckwheat groats (pre-cook in water and
>   sauerkraut juice)
> pinch of sea salt
> 2 Tbsp finely chopped parsley
> 1 cup steamed, chopped kale or leftover leafy greens
> 1 cup chopped, drained sauerkraut
> ½ cup red cabbage, thinly sliced, blanched and sprinkled with
>   ¼ tsp brown rice vinegar to brighten and preserve the color

¼ to ½ cup soy sauce
1 tsp ginger juice

Sauté finely chopped parsley in a very small amount of water. Mix the parsley with the buckwheat. Mix in the steamed, chopped kale and chopped sauerkraut. Mix the soy sauce and ginger juice, pour over the buckwheat salad, and mix in.

TABOULI SALAD
Yield: 4½ cups

This is a variation from *Book of Whole Meals* by Annemarie Colbin, page 192. (See: *www.foodandhealing.com*)

1½ cups water
1 cup bulgur
Mint dressing:
  2 Tbsp lemon juice
  1 Tbsp soy sauce
  2 Tbsp olive oil
  5 leaves fresh mint, 2 Tbsp
  1 handful parsley, ½ cup
  1 stalk celery, ¾ cup
  3 whole scallions, ½ cup
  5 med radishes, ¼ cup
  5 large Romaine lettuce leaves
  alfalfa sprouts

To prepare bulgur, add 1½ cups boiling water to 1 cup bulgur. Cover and let sit 45 minutes or until water is absorbed. Fluff—will yield about 3 cups cooked bulgur.

To make mint dressing: Combine lemon juice, soy sauce, and olive oil in a small bowl or jar, mixing well. Chop the mint very fine and add to the liquid mixture. To improve the flavor, allow the dressing to stand for 10 to 15 minutes.

Chop the parsley, celery, and scallion; slice the radishes into thin rounds. Combine the vegetables in a salad bowl and stir in the bulgur. Add the Mint Dressing, toss and allow to marinate for 45 minutes. Serve on lettuce leaves topped with sprouts.

For additional grain recipes, see:

Crackers—Packy Conway, page 79.

Cumin-Scented Quinoa with Shiitake Mushroom Sauce—Meredith McCarty, page 93.

Fresh Herb Couscous—Laura Stec, page 106.

Mixed Media Summer Salad—Ginat Rice, page 104.

Nappa Cabbage Quinoa Rolls with Sesame Sauce—Susanne Jensen, page 88.

Pot Stickers—Susanne Jensen, page 86.

Rice Croquettes—Yvette DeLangre, page 83.

Spicy Udon Salad—Barb Jurecki-Humphrey, page 91.

Soba Summer Salad—David and Cynthia Briscoe, page 66.

Tamales, and Arepas—Dawn Pallavi, page 98.

The Only Main Course Salad Recipe You Need—Rebecca Wood, page 119.

Three Grain Pilaf—Laura Stec, page 108.

Wayfarer's Bread—Rebecca Wood, page 120.

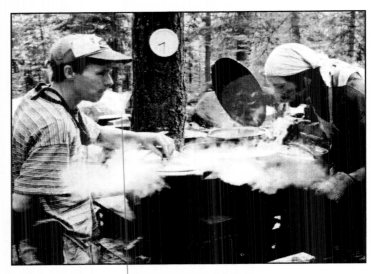

James and Tosh Cooking at the 2002 French Meadows Camp

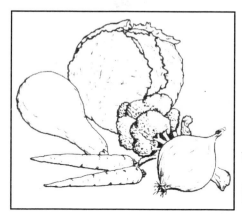

Vegetables at Every Meal

Vegetables are colorful, delicious, and plentiful at French Meadows camp. They appear in salads, freshly cooked side dishes, and dishes with grains, sea vegetables, or miso. Every meal has vegetables; even breakfasts, as the staff serves vegetables from the previous night's dinner. Preparing vegetables at camp is similar to preparing them at home, with the exception that there is no refrigeration at camp—everything must be planned and coordinated to use while fresh so there is no waste.

Green vegetables are served daily at camp and coordinated with freshness in mind. Salads are served the first few days and immediately after the vegetable delivery while lettuce is in its prime. Kale, leafy greens, and broccoli are prepared also. Green cabbage and Chinese cabbage and bok choy last a few days longer. At home in the refrigerator, a similar thing happens; cabbage lasts longer in the crisper than lettuce or broccoli.

The recipes that follow are some of the favorites served at camp. They reflect summer's bounty and cooking preparation and can easily be used other times of the year.

Solo Vegetables

Certain vegetables such as corn on the cob or winter squash are best when cooked and served singly. Other vegetables are enhanced through cooking separately even though they are served together. This type of cooking is useful when blanching vegetables, as timing is crucial and varies with different kinds of vegetables. After cooking, serve vegetables alongside a full meal, or mix with other vegetables in a salad or to top noodles.

CORN ON THE COB

Yield: 4 pieces

> **½ cup water**
> **¼ tsp sea salt**
> **2 large ears of corn, broken or cut into 4-inch pieces**

Bring water to a boil. Add sea salt. Add corn, cover, and bring to a boil. Simmer 7 to 10 minutes until tender. If desired, dab a pinch of umeboshi paste on corn while eating.

WINTER SQUASH

Yield: 4 cups

> **1 cup water**
> **½ large butternut squash, washed, seeded, and cut into 2-inch**
> **squares, 5 cups**
> **¼ tsp sea salt**

Place water in a pan. Place squash on top and sprinkle sea salt on top. Cover and bring to a boil. Simmer 30 minutes or until tender. Gently remove while serving to retain shape.

BLANCHING VEGETABLES

Many vegetables are blanched at camp because it is easier when preparing quantities of food. At home, preparation is simplified due to smaller amounts and also, due to lower elevation. Water boils at a lower temperature at 5000 feet and thus vegetables require more cooking time to become tender.

When blanching, time carefully for best results. Some vegetables, such as shredded Chinese Cabbage require 15 to 20 seconds of immersion. Others, such as green beans can take as long as 8 minutes. Timing depends on the age of the vegetable, whether or not the vegetable is cut, and the thickness of the pieces.

The following procedure gives a description of how to blanch and uses vegetables that are prepared at camp with suggested timings for the home kitchen. Use your own experience to prepare vegetables according to your liking.

Blanching Procedure: Bring water to a boil. Use enough water to completely submerge vegetables while cooking; use a large enough pot to allow room for expansion. For example, use 8 cups of water for 1 bunch of kale; use 4 cups of water for ¼ pound of snow peas.

When water boils, add salt if used. Use salt for all vegetables except leafy greens. Salt brings out more flavor for vegetables; for leafy greens, salt can increase bitterness. In addition, blanching leafy greens removes some of the bitterness and they taste better. Blanching is the preferred method for preparing kale, collards, mustard greens, and other greens that become bitter when sautéed or steamed.

Add vegetables, one kind at a time, and without covering pan, return to a boil. Cook to desired texture, crisp or tender. Remove with a slotted spoon or strainer. Drain in colander and separate gently to cool. Cook a second vegetable if desired. After all vegetables are cool, serve or mix with other vegetables and dressings as desired. After blanching, use cooking water to cook pasta, or save for soup, if not bitter.

Broccoli—Use salt. Cut each stalk 3 inches below flower; separate into flowerets. (Save stems for use in soup.) When water comes to a boil, add broccoli, stem side down. Return to a boil, then immediately, remove and drain. Broccoli retains crispness. If you wish tenderer broccoli, boil 1 to 2 minutes.

Snow peas—Use salt. Trim stems off snow peas. When water boils, add snow peas and simmer 3 to 4 minutes. Remove and drain.

Kale, radish greens, or baby bok choy—Avoid salt. Prepare greens well: discard wilted or discolored leaves, remove hard stems on kale, and wash well in a basin of water to remove sand. Cut into shreds or tear into bite size pieces. When water boils, immerse one of these kinds of greens and time as follows: kale 1 to 2 minutes, up to 5 if thick; radish greens, 30 seconds to 1 minute; baby bok choy, 1 to 2 minutes, up to 5 minutes. Baby bok choy can be separated into stalks and leaves. Blanch separately: stalks up to 5 minutes and leaves for 1 to 2 minutes.

Green beans and carrots—Use salt. Cook one kind at a time. Cut green beans into 2-inch lengths and blanch for 5 to 8 minutes. Cut carrots into matchstick pieces, similar in size to green beans. Blanch for 4 to 5 minutes. After cooking, mix and serve together.

BOILED SALAD
Yield: 5 cups

>   6 cups water
>   ¼ tsp sea salt
>   ½ Chinese cabbage, shredded, 5 cups
>   1 med carrot, thin matchsticks, ¾ cup
>   Dressing: 1 Tbsp umeboshi vinegar and 3 Tbsp olive oil

Bring water to a boil. Add salt. Blanch Chinese cabbage for 15 to 20 seconds, then remove. Add carrot and blanch 1 to 2 minutes. Remove. When vegetables are cooled, mix with dressing and serve.

Mixed Vegetables

Mixed vegetable dishes can be simple or ornate. The sautéed vegetables listed here are a step-up from the solo vegetables, utilizing onion in the dishes with the respective vegetable. Onion adds sweetness to vegetable dishes, especially when sautéed. The Arame and carrot dish includes arame sea vegetable, and the Onion miso dish adds miso. The Chunky pasta sauce adds herbs. Also included are two grain and vegetable combination dishes. The Noodle and Vegetable Dish is a full meal. The Cauliflower and Millet "Mashed Potatoes" is served with Seitan and Sage Gravy as printed in the protein chapter.

CROOKNECK SQUASH AND ONIONS
Yield: 5 cups

>   1 tsp light sesame oil or olive oil
>   1 med onion, thin crescents, 1½ cups
>   8 med yellow squash, cut into chunks, 8 cups
>   ½ to 1 tsp sea salt

Heat oil in a pan. Sauté onion with a pinch of sea salt until transparent. Add squash and the rest of the sea salt and sauté 1 to 2 minutes. Stir constantly. Cover. (If you have a otoshibuta, a Japanese "drop cover", moisten and place directly on top of squash in pan; then cover pan with lid. This kind of cover is made of wood but can be substituted with a small lid. It fits inside the cooking pan and traps heat close to the vegetables. Vegetables release more of their own juices, and flavor sweetens.) Simmer vegetables over low heat for about 20 minutes, stirring once or twice. Vegetables will simmer in their own juices.

CABBAGE AND ONIONS
Yield: 3 cups

> **1 tsp light sesame oil or olive oil**
> **1 med onion, thin crescents, 1½ cups**
> **½ med cabbage; 5 cups**
> > **core, finely minced**
> > **leaves, 1-inch squares**
> **½ tsp sea salt**
> **½ tsp ume vinegar**

Cook cabbage in the same manner as listed above for yellow squash. Add ume vinegar at the end of cooking to season.

ARAME AND CARROT
Yield: 3 cups

> **1 cup arame, soaked in 2 cups water, will swell to 2 cups**
> **1 onion, thin crescents, 2 cups**
> **1 carrot, thin matchsticks, 1 cup**
> **1 to 2 tsp light sesame oil**
> **2 Tbsp soy sauce**

Soak arame for 5 to 10 minutes. Drain and reserve soaking water. Rinse again. Measure. If you have more or less than 2 cups of arame, adjust the soy sauce quantity accordingly.

Heat oil in a pan. Add onion and sauté until transparent. Add carrots and sauté. Add 1 cup of reserved soaking water. Lay arame on top. Add soy sauce. Bring to a boil and simmer 20 to 25 minutes. Remove cover and cook away remaining liquid. Sea palm and hijiki are prepared in similar manner and can be substituted for arame in this recipe.

ONION MISO
Yield: 3 cups

>**2 tsp light sesame oil**
>**4 med onions, thin crescents, 6 cups**
>**¼ tsp sea salt**
>**2 Tbsp water**
>**2 to 4 tsp soybean, barley, and/or rice miso**

Heat oil. Sauté onion with sea salt until transparent, 1 to 2 minutes. Add water, cover and bring to a boil. (Otoshibuta can be used here.) Simmer over low heat 10 to 15 minutes until onion is tender. Add miso in small pats on top on onions. Cover and simmer 5 minutes to soften miso. Stir miso into onion.

NOODLE AND VEGETABLE DISH
Yield 8 servings

>**4 quarts water**
>**½ bunch kale, remove hard stems, cut leaves into bite-sized**
>**   squares, 4 cups**
>**½ tsp sea salt**
>**½ pound green beans, cut into 2-inch lengths, 2 cups**
>**1 pound Eden garlic ribbons, or other pasta**
>**1 Tbsp light sesame oil**
>**1 onion, thin crescents, 2 cups**
>**½ tsp sea salt**
>**¼ Chinese cabbage, cut into 1-inch pieces, 3 cups**
>**2 med yellow squash, chunks, 2 cups**
>**1 carrot, thin matchsticks, 1 cup**
>**Dressing**—Yield: 2 cups
>**2 cups walnuts**
>**4 Tbsp soy sauce**
>**1 cup boiling water**

In large pasta pot, bring water to a boil. Blanch kale, boiling for up to 5 minutes; remove and drain. Add sea salt (to the same water) and blanch the green beans. Boil 5 to 8 minutes or until tender; remove and drain. In the same water, add the garlic ribbons. Bring to a boil and simmer 7 to 10 minutes until *al dente*. Drain, rinse, and drain again.

In the meantime, heat oil in a pan and sauté the onion with a pinch of salt until transparent. Add Chinese cabbage, yellow squash and carrot, one kind at a time and sauté 1 to 2 minutes before adding the next vegetable. Add the rest of the salt. Cover and simmer over low heat for 7 to 10 minutes until tender, stirring once or twice. Vegetables will cook in own juices. Use otoshibuta if desired.

To make the dressing: roast the walnuts in a dry skillet, stirring often, from 5 to 7 minutes. Place in blender with soy sauce and boiling water and process until smooth. If blender is small, process in two batches. Serve noodles with vegetables and dressing on top.

CHUNKY PASTA SAUCE
Yield: 4 cups

>1 tsp light sesame oil
>1 med onion, crescents, 1½ cups
>½ to ¾ cup water
>½ small butternut squash, seeded, cut into 1-inch squares, 2 cups
>3 med carrots, large chunks, 2 cups
>1 bay leaf
>1½ tsp oregano
>1½ tsp basil
>½ tsp sea salt

Heat oil. Sauté onion with a pinch of sea salt until transparent. Add water, squash, and carrots. Sprinkle herbs and sea salt on top. Bring to a boil and simmer 25 to 30 minutes until tender. Mash to a chunky consistency and serve on pasta.

CAULIFLOWER AND MILLET "MASHED POTATOES"
Yield: 5 cups

>3 cups water
>¼ tsp sea salt
>1 cup millet, rinsed and drained
>½ med cauliflower, chopped, 2 cups

Boil water in a 3 or 4 quart pan. Add sea salt and millet. Cover and return to a boil. Add cauliflower, cover pan and simmer 30 minutes over low heat, using a heat diffuser if needed. There is no need to stir. When cauliflower is tender and water is absorbed, remove from heat and mash together.

For additional vegetable recipes, see

Burdock Ribs—Packy Conway, page 77.

Carrot Tofu Aspic—David and Cynthia Briscoe, page 67.

Grated Carrot Salad with Sweet Rice Vinegar—Ginat Rice, page 104.

Greens with Grated Beet and Orange—Susanne Jensen, page 85.

Grilled Vegetables—Laura Stec, page 107.

Hiziki Side Dish—Yvette DeLangre, page 83.

Organic Field Green Salad with Candied Almonds and Sweet Mustard-Garlic Vinaigrette—Meredith McCarty, page 95.

Oven-Roasted Winter Root Vegetables—Laura Stec, page 106.

Parsnip Delight—Bob Carr, page 70.

Quick-and-Easy Tangy Cole Slaw—Bob Carr, page 72.

Season's Greens and Red Radishes with Citrus-Flax Oil Vinaigrette—Meredith McCarty, page 95.

Steamed Kabocha Salad—David and Cynthia Briscoe, page 69.

Stir-Fried Vegetables—Yvette DeLangre, page 82.

Wakame Cucumber Salad—Ginat Rice, page 105.

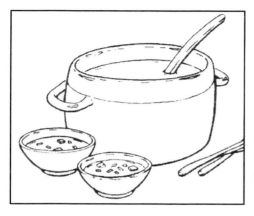

Favorite Camp Soups

Savory. Sweet. Soothing. Soups have a way of satisfying the palette as well as the stomach. Simple or ornate and appropriate in any season, soup is valued in all cuisines—both sensually and nutritionally.

Soup can be a main course, a side dish, or a simple broth to flavor noodles. It can be warming in cool times and soft and moist in hot times. Various vegetables, beans, grains, or pastas and seasonings such as miso, soy sauce, or herbs give rise to an abundant array of soups.

Soup is unique in that it fits anywhere on any food pyramid. Soup can be considered a carbohydrate source when grains are used, a protein source when beans or beans and grains in combination are included, and a fat source when oil is used to sauté ingredients.

Many soups are characterized by the choice of vegetables. Seasonal availability dictates fresh corn in soups in the summer or winter squash in soups in the winter. Other vegetables such as onions, celery, or garlic flavor soups at any time of the year.

Whether at home, eating out, or camping, soups have a place at the table. Most of the following soups are prepared each summer at the French Meadows camp. Each year campers request recipes so they can cook them at home. Although served at camp in the summer, these recipes aren't limited to the hot time of the year. It is easy to change recipes by substituting ingredients; increasing or decreasing the amount of miso, oil, or water; or by serving the soup at a temperature suited for the day. See the comments under each heading to vary recipes based on your needs and the time of year. Hopefully, they will become your favorites, too.

Miso Soup

Soup is served daily at French Meadows camp. Cornellia Aihara, creator of the original camp menus, served miso soup every lunch when she was head cook. This tradition continues under co-head cooks, Packy Conway and Suzanne Jensen. Camp is warm at noon, so ingredients usually include cabbage, summer squash, and other summer vegetables. The miso soup recipe included here contains hearty vegetables appropriate for cooler temperatures and is not actually served at camp. Turnips aren't included in the camp inventory as they are often bitter in summer. The recipe may be altered for any time of year by substituting vegetables of choice in similar quantities.

Cornellia taught me how to make miso soup and stressed the importance of using wakame and of sautéing the vegetables. This method can be used with other vegetables and is suitable year-round.

HEARTY WINTER MISO SOUP
Yield: 8 cups

> 6-inch strip of wakame, soaked in 2 cups water;
>> stems, thin rounds
>> leaves, ½-inch squares
> 1 tsp light sesame oil
> 1 large onion, thin crescents, 2 cups
> ½ small butternut squash, ½-inch squares, 2 cups
> 2 small turnips, diced, 1 cup
> 1½ cups reserved soaking water
> 4 cups boiling water
> 2 Tbsp barley miso

Soak wakame in cold water until soft, 10 to 15 minutes. Drain and reserve soaking water. Separate leaves from stems and cut each as directed. Heat oil in a pan and sauté onion until transparent. Add vegetables in the order listed, one kind at a time. Sauté each kind until fragrant, 1 to 2 minutes. Place wakame stems on top of the vegetables. Add reserved soaking water and boiling water, using care not to disturb layers. Cover and bring to a boil. Simmer 20 to 25 minutes. Add wakame leaves and simmer another 5 minutes. Dilute miso with ¼ cup of the hot broth and then mix with soup. Heat through but do not boil.

Vegetable Soups

Vegetable soups are delicious and provide a visual and nutritional accompaniment to a meal of grains and beans. The following two soups are always favorites at camp.

CREAMY ONION SOUP
Yield: 9 cups

This recipe is prepared with or without oatmeal depending on the weather of the day—oatmeal produces a warming creamy soup.

> **1 tsp light sesame oil**
> **2 med onions, thin crescents, 3 cups**
> **2 large celery stalks, thin diagonals, 1½ cups**
> **8 cups boiling water**
> **1 cup rolled oats or 2 cups cooked oatmeal**
> **¼ teaspoon sea salt**
> **1½ to 2 Tbsp rice miso**

Heat oil in a pan and sauté onion with a pinch of salt until transparent. Add celery and sauté briefly. Add boiling water. Place rolled oats (or cooked oatmeal) on top. Sprinkle remaining salt on top of the grain. Cover. Bring to a boil. Simmer 30 minutes with the lid ajar to prevent foaming over. Dilute miso in a small amount of the broth before seasoning the whole pot; or alternately, if you won't be eating the whole pot at once, season individual bowls.

CORN CHOWDER
Yield: 11 cups

This recipe is a variation from *Natural Foods Cookbook* by Mary Estella, page 112. It relies on cornmeal or polenta to thicken the soup. Many recipes for corn chowder use arrowroot powder to produce a translucent soup base, whereas polenta produces a creamy soup base.

At camp, polenta is a useful choice over arrowroot powder. Since this recipe is expanded 10 times, polenta provides a reliable and more cost-effective thickening agent than arrowroot. In the home kitchen, either one provides satisfactory results. If desired, omit polenta and use arrowroot in this recipe: Cook soup as per recipe until tender; dissolve 5 tablespoons of arrowroot powder in ½ cup cold water; and add to soup to thicken, stirring constantly until translucent.

> **6 ears corn, cut off cob, 4 cups**
> **1 strip kombu (optional)**
> **8 cups water**
> **1 tsp light sesame oil**
> **1 large onion, diced, 2 cups**
> **1 stalk of celery, diced, ¾ cup**
> **½ cup cornmeal or polenta**
> **1 to 2 Tbsp white miso or sea salt to taste**
> **Garnish: dill or basil, chopped**

Slice corn off cob. Make stock: place cobs and kombu in pot; add water; simmer 15 minutes. In a large soup pot, sauté onion and celery in oil over medium-low heat. Add corn. Sprinkle cornmeal or polenta in and stir well so vegetables are coated with it. When it begins to turn golden, strain corncob from hot stock and add stock to vegetables, stirring quickly to prevent lumps. Place pot on heat diffuser; lower heat and simmer for one-half hour. Dissolve miso in water and add to soup before serving. Adjust saltiness to taste with miso or sea salt and garnish with chopped dill or basil.

Bean Soups

Bean soups disappear at camp. No matter how much the kitchen prepares, none is left over.

MINESTRONE SOUP
Yield: 4 servings (5 cups)

The minestrone soup doubles as a miso soup and is varied at camp with the substitution of onion for scallion. It originates from *American Macrobiotic Cuisine* by Meredith McCarty, page 21.

¼ **cup small white navy beans**
3-inch piece kombu
5 cups water (2 cups to cook beans, 3 cups more for soup)
2 cloves garlic, minced
½ **cup carrot, diced small**
½ **cup cabbage, diced small**
½ **cup celery, diced small**
½ **cup scallions, diced small**
½ **cup pasta**
2 to 3 Tbsp barley (mugi) miso
2 Tbsp parsley, chopped

Soak beans with kombu in two cups water for 6 to 8 hours. Cover and bring to pressure to cook one-half hour. Remove kombu from pot and dice. Return to soup with three cups more water, pasta, and vegetables (except parsley). Return soup to boil and slow boil until done, about 15 minutes.

Dissolve miso in a little of the hot soup broth and add to soup with parsley. Cook three minutes more over very low heat to blend flavors.

Vary the vegetables according to season. Summer squash is a nice addition during the warm months.

Pea Soup

Yield: 10 cups

Pea soup is prepared at camp in a traditional manner and is served with crackers and peanut butter for a simple and satisfying meal.

2 cups green split peas
10 cups water
1 large onion, minced, 2 cups
2 med celery stalks, quarter rounds, 1½ cups
2 med carrots, thin quarter rounds, 1½ cups
optional spices: garlic, bay leaf
½ **tsp salt**
5 tsp soy sauce, optional

Wash peas and drain. Cover and bring to a boil in water. Simmer for 50 to 60 minutes until soft. Add vegetables. Sprinkle sea salt on top. Return to a boil and simmer 30 minutes over low heat, using a heat diffuser, if needed. Add soy sauce, if used.

BLACK BEAN SOUP
Yield: 10 cups

This soup is enhanced with the addition of seitan. Cooked seitan chunks are added to the soup immediately before serving and can be added to this recipe if desired. The recipe for Seitan is in the Protein chapter, page 37. With or without seitan, this recipe is delicious served any time of year.

> **2 cups black beans**
> **4 inches kombu**
> **4 to 6 cups water**
> **1 teaspoon light sesame oil**
> **1 large onion, minced, 2 cups**
> **2 to 3 cloves garlic, finely minced**
> **1 stalk celery, thin quarter rounds, 1 cup**
> **1 large carrot, thin half rounds, 1 cup**
> **½ tsp cumin or more**
> **¼ tsp coriander or more**
> **2 Tbsp parsley, finely minced**
> **2 Tbsp cilantro, finely minced**
> **4 cups additional water**
> **½ tsp salt**
> **2 cups cooked seitan, cut into chunks, optional, page 37**

Soak black turtle beans with kombu for 6 to 8 hours, using 6 cups of water if boiling or 4 cups of water if pressure cooking. Boil for 1½ to 2 hours or pressure cook for 45 minutes until beans are tender.

In another pot, sauté onion until transparent. Add vegetables in order listed, one kind at a time. Sauté each kind for 1 to 2 minutes. Add spices. Sauté briefly to enhance flavor. Add additional water. Layer beans and bean cooking water on top. Sprinkle sea salt on top of the beans. Cover and bring to a boil. Simmer 30 minutes on low heat. Add cooked seitan, if using, after this time. Serve.

Broth for Soba

This broth is a traditional Japanese recipe that is simple to make and a powerhouse of nutrition. Kombu seaweed with or without shiitake mushrooms is used to make "dashi"—a stock rich in the minerals and rejuvenating properties of seaweed. Flavored with soy sauce, it accompanies cooked soba well. Garnish with chopped scallions to serve.

KOMBU CLEAR SOUP, WITH OR WITHOUT SHIITAKE MUSHROOM
Yield: 4 cups

> **4-inch piece of kombu**
> **2 dried shiitake mushrooms, optional**
> **4 cups cold water**
> **4 Tbsp soy sauce**

Place kombu and shiitake mushrooms, if used, in cold water. Cover pan and bring to a rolling boil. Remove kombu and shiitake mushrooms immediately. Add soy sauce. Leftover kombu can be cooked with beans. Leftover Kombu Clear Soup With Shiitake Mushrooms can be used in Kombu and Shiitake Condiment, page 45.

For additional soup recipes, see

Carrot Lime Soup—Susanne Jensen, page 85.

Cauliflower Curry Coconut Soup—Barb Jurecki-Humphrey, page 90.

Chickpea Stew—Lenore Baum, page 63.

Minestrone Soup—Packy Conway, page 78.

Red Lentil Corn Chowder—Lenore Baum, page 64.

Three Sister Soup—Rebecca Wood, page 118.

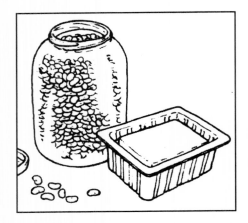

Protein at Camp and Home

Protein at camp is plentiful. It is present in a variety of ways such as seeds at breakfast, tofu at lunch, and black bean soup for dinner. It is served at the first meal and the last. Next to complex carbohydrates, protein has a prominent place on every plate.

Protein is needed for health and adds to the feeling of satisfaction. Nutritionally, protein helps the body grow. Adequate nutrition is required in all stages of macrobiotic practice, whether one is new to this way of eating, or has eaten so for years. The following recipes are served at camp and in my home kitchen. They are always requested.

Seitan

Seitan (SAY tahn) is a product made from wheat gluten that is high in protein. It can be used in soups, stews, casseroles, stir-fries, or served on its own.

Different recipes use various combinations of whole-wheat flour and water to make dough, sometimes including white flour and gluten flour. The dough is washed—as one would wash clothing—to extract the starch and bran, leaving a glutinous ball half as large as the original dough. The gluten ball is cut into pieces and simmered in broth to make seitan; the starch and bran can be saved for other uses. Seitan is not difficult to make, but it does require time and a lot of water.

This recipe was designed for camp using gluten flour only—the starch and bran already have been removed—to save time for the busy cooks. Since there is no starch or bran, there is no need to wash the dough with water, which is wasteful for a forest environment. Seasonings are added to the dough directly to add more flavors.

Use quality products in production, such as extra virgin and organic unrefined olive oil and coconut oil in the dough and for frying. Gluten flour is available in natural food stores.

In addition to the uses below, seitan (unfried) is added to black bean soup at camp; see page 34. Seitan is also delicious added to stir-fried vegetables, mixed with cooked pasta and sauce, or sautéed with onions and green peppers to make seitan fajita. Feel free to experiment by adding seitan to your favorite dishes.

SEITAN CUTLETS
Yield: 6 cups

> **2 cups gluten flour**
> **1 tsp granulated garlic**
> **2 tsp granulated onion**
> **1 tsp ground cumin**
> **2 Tbsp olive oil**
> **¼ cup soy sauce**
> **1 Tbsp ginger juice**
> **1 ¼ cups water**
> **Broth**
> > **4 cups water**
> > **¼ cup soy sauce**

Mix gluten flour with spices; mix liquid ingredients. Mix well together and knead briefly. Let sit 30 minutes.

In a 6-quart pan, heat water to a boil, and add soy sauce. Cut or tear gluten into pieces, large or small. Gently lower into broth. Return to boil and simmer 30 minutes over gentle heat. Seitan will expand during cooking and then condense some when cooled.

FRIED SEITAN
Slice drained and cooked seitan into ¼-inch thick pieces. Prepare a coating of arrowroot powder, or a mixture of arrowroot powder and

gomashio, or arrowroot and ground flax seeds. Dip each piece in coating. Heat coconut oil in skillet. Pan-fry slices until crispy, 3 to 4 minutes each side.

SAGE GRAVY

Yield: 2½ cups

This gravy is served on top of the seitan at camp alongside "Millet Mashed Potatoes"—a dish made of millet cooked with cauliflower page 27.

> **1 tsp olive oil**
> **1 onion, minced, 1½ cups**
> **1 Tbsp minced garlic**
> **1 tsp sage leaf**
> **1 Tbsp thyme leaf**
> **1 cup broth from cooking seitan**
> **½ cup tahini**
> **½ cup water**
> **1 Tbsp arrowroot powder**
> **1 to 2 tsp soy sauce, to taste**

Heat oil, sauté onion until transparent, add garlic and herbs, and sauté briefly to release fragrance. Add broth, heat to a boil, and simmer 5 minutes. Mix tahini, water, arrowroot, and 1 teaspoon of soy sauce. Add to pan and heat until thickened. Taste and adjust seasonings. Serve on top of cooked seitan; or, add 1 cup diced seitan cubes to sauce and serve.

Tofu

Tofu is more popular than ever these days, making an appearance not only in water-packed containers in natural food stores, but also in aseptic and vacuum-sealed packages in major grocery stores. Buy the best tofu you can find: organic, made from non-GMO (genetically modified organisms) soybeans, and natural nigari. The better the tofu, the better this recipe turns out. If you have a choice, choose hard-style tofu over soft-style varieties for fried tofu.

FRIED TOFU
Yield: 12 pieces

 1 pound tofu
 coconut oil for frying
 Marinade
 3 Tbsp soy sauce
 1 Tbsp ginger juice
 1 Tbsp roasted sesame oil
 Coating
 4 Tbsp gomashio
 4 Tbsp arrowroot powder

Slice tofu into ¼- to ½-inch-thick rectangular pieces. Remove excess water by pressing between two flat surfaces, such as two cutting boards. Paper toweling under the tofu will speed the process. Weight with a heavy pan or a bottle of water for 5 minutes. Remove.

To marinate: place tofu in marinade for 3 to 4 hours, turning occasionally until the marinade is absorbed. Tofu can marinade in refrigerator overnight if desired.

To fry: prepare coating. Dip each piece in coating. Heat oil in skillet. Pan-fry tofu until golden, 3 to 4 minutes on each side.

Alternately, if there is no time to marinade: Press tofu as above to remove excess water. Prepare coating, dip tofu in coating, and pan fry. Use marinade ingredients as a dipping sauce after frying.

LENTIL PÂTÉ
Yield: 3 cups

Lentil pâté is often baked. This recipe is prepared on the stovetop as there are no ovens at camp. The resulting dish is thick enough to serve on top of crackers.

 1 cup lentils
 3 cups water
 ½ onion, diced, ¾ cup
 1 stalk celery, diced, ¾ cup
 ¼ tsp sea salt
 garlic, curry powder, thyme leaf
 1 Tbsp tahini
 1 Tbsp soy sauce

Soak lentils in water, if desired, for 1 to 2 hours. Bring to a boil and simmer 40 minutes until soft, adding extra water if needed to prevent scorching. Add cut vegetables, spices, and sea salt. Cover and bring to a boil. Simmer 30 minutes over low heat with heat diffuser if necessary. Add tahini and soy sauce and mash or purée in a food processor. Serve on rye crackers.

AZUKI BEANS WITH WINTER SQUASH
Yield: 4½ cups

Azuki beans with squash is a standard macrobiotic recipe—azuki beans, winter squash, and seaweed combine in taste and nutrition. According to Marc Van Cauwenberghe, M.D., in *Macrobiotic Home Remedies* (page 57), this dish can help regulate blood sugar levels, boost vitality, and strengthen the kidneys. Cornellia Aihara states in *Natural Healing from Head to Toe* that this dish is useful for many illnesses including heart disorders and nervous system malfunction (page 206). If squash has an especially hard outer skin, peel before simmering with the beans.

> **1 cup azuki beans**
> **3 cups water**
> **2 inches kombu**
> **½ large butternut squash, 1-inch squares, 4 cups**
> **¼ tsp sea salt**

Soak azuki beans with kombu for 4 to 6 hours. Bring to a boil and simmer 45 minutes until soft, adding extra water if needed to prevent scorching. After 45 minutes, add squash and sprinkle salt on top. Return to a boil. Simmer 30 minutes over low heat, using a heat diffuser if needed until squash is tender. Mix to serve.

For additional protein recipes, see:
Bean Soups—pages 29-35.
Black Bean Salsa—Susanne Jensen, page 86.
Braised Tempeh with Green Herb Coulis—Meredith McCarty, page 96.
Chickpea Stew—Lenore Baum, page 63.
Italian White Bean Hummus—Susanne Jensen, page 84.
Pinto Beans and Onions—Susanne Jensen, page 86.
Red Lentil Corn Chowder—Lenore Baum, page 64.
Tamales—Dawn Pallavi, page 98.
Tempeh Mochi Reuben—Barb Jurecki-Humphrey, page 89.
Tempeh, Mushroom, and Celery Fricassee—Laura Stec, page 107.
White Beans Vinaigrette—Annemarie Colbin, page 75.

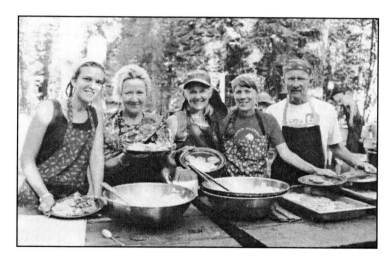

Beth, Kaja, Barb, Noel, and David Serving Lunch at the 2004 French Meadows Camp

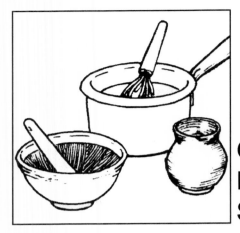

Condiments, Dressings, and Side Dishes

Condiments are to brown rice what dressings are to salads and side dishes are to meals—that is—the adornment. Like butter to bread or salsa to chips, condiments, dressings, and side dishes are a natural extension—the finishing touch that boosts flavor, peaks color, and supplies additional complement.

Condiments, dressings, and side dishes are more than just a perk. They can be used to create another dimension to meals—the dimension of balance. Balance in meals is more than just the presence of complex carbohydrates, complete proteins, and quality fats. Balance is more than aligning foods and techniques with the season. Balance includes the theory of energetics, the ideas of yin and yang in sync with the season, one's personal health, and the choices of foods and preparation styles in order to enhance one's well being. It need not be hit and miss to be healthy. It can be a conscious choice—a choice that involves commonsense ideas with the inclusion of specific foods for support.

Macrobiotic teaching emphasizes the need to "lighten" up for summer by utilizing fresh foods and less cooking. Summer is hot—a yang time of year—so the advice is to avoid excess yang and to incorporate quality yin things. It is often taught that one needs to avoid excess heaviness such as concentrated foods or dishes high in fat and/or salt. I do this through choosing salads over long-cooked vegetable dishes, serving a higher percentage of vegetables to grains, and preparing grains and beans in the morning before the day gets really hot.

When I began macrobiotics I was under the impression that one should use less miso, soy sauce, salt, and oil in the summer in order to fit with the idea of "lightening"—the theory that salty foods and frying in oil are "too yangizing" for summer. Imagine my shock when I saw Cornellia Aihara preparing oily miso condiment, a dish consisting of oil and miso with a tad of water or lemon juice, in the summer. Why such a heavy yang dish in the hot time of year?

Cornellia told me that when the season turns hot, it is very tempting to eat a lot of fruit or drink a lot of juices or beer—items that if taken in excess can be depleting or weakening, or in her words, "too yin." One must learn how to use foods to create vitality in the summer, or as she said, "strong cooking is needed in summer too." She felt oily miso was such an energy-providing dish, and she would prepare it at all times of the year or for special need. For instance, after I delivered my second baby, she made a batch of oily miso to help me in the recovery. Oily miso provides good-quality oil in combination with good-quality miso. It is served one-half to one teaspoon on top of a thick round of boiled daikon or raw cucumber, depending on season, and is pleasing in taste, presentation, and yin-yang balance.

Miso, umeboshi, and soy sauce are concentrated foods and when used in condiments, dressings, and side dishes, one can benefit from their strength while not having to make the entire meal too salty or heavy. Remember that salt is needed in summer. If we drink more water in the summer, which is a good idea when active, outside a lot, or living in a dry climate, we are naturally "lightening" through carrying more water volume; salt is necessary to maintain the sodium/potassium ratio in the blood. In addition, we perspire more in the summer and need to replace the salt that is eliminated.

The following condiments, dressings, and side dishes provide a quality factor to meals. Miso, umeboshi, and soy sauce provide quality salt. Olive oil, sesame oil, and tahini provide quality fat. Sea vegetables provide quality minerals.

All of these recipes are served at camp with a full menu of grains, beans, and vegetables.

Condiments

The following three condiments are flavorful and powerful—a little goes a long ways.

Oily Miso

Yield: ¼ cup

This and the following recipe are served at camp at the same meal with a variety of other items—pea soup, crackers and peanut butter, brown rice, cooked cabbage, and cucumbers. This recipe is served on top of rounds of boiled daikon radish.

> **1 Tbsp sesame oil**
> **3 Tbsp dark miso, such as barley miso**
> **1 Tbsp lemon juice**

Heat oil. Add miso. Sauté until fragrant, 1 to 2 minutes, stirring constantly to smooth lumps. Add liquid gradually, thinning to desired consistency.

Nori Condiment

Yield: 1½ cups

This condiment has an unusual appearance and is usually greeted with a surprise and a question as to what it is. It looks like mush; yet the flavor is delicious and it is devoured—none is leftover. It is served alongside the other dishes.

> **10 sheets nori**
> **2 cups water**
> **4 to 5 tsp soy sauce**

Tear nori into 1-inch squares. Soak in water for 10 to 15 minutes. Add soy sauce, cover pan, and bring to a boil. Simmer over low heat for 15 minutes. Serve 1 to 2 tablespoons per serving. This will keep for a week stored in the refrigerator.

Note: To serve this condiment with other menus, choose dishes with a variety of texture and colors—brown rice, chickpeas, blanched broccoli, and almonds; or udon, onion soup, scrambled tofu, and crisp salad.

KOMBU AND SHIITAKE CONDIMENT

Yield: ¼ cup

This condiment is made at camp after first making clear soup to serve with soba noodles. See page 35.

4-inch piece kombu, reserved from making soup
2 shiitake mushrooms, reserved from making soup
1 cup water
1½ tsp soy sauce

Cut kombu into very thin matchsticks. Discard the stem from shiitake and slice the cap into thin crescents. Add the cut kombu and shiitake mushrooms to water and soy sauce. Cover pan, bring to a boil, and simmer 30 minutes over low heat. Remove lid and boil away any remaining liquid.

To make this condiment without first making soup, soak kombu and shiitake mushrooms prior to cutting. Soak separately, each in 1 cup of water for 15 to 25 minutes. Drain, reserve soaking water, and then proceed as above, using the reserved soaking water to cook the condiment.

Dressings

The following three dressings include umeboshi plums or umeboshi vinegar. Umeboshi is a tonic in summer, providing digestive strength for the body and a refreshing taste in addition to green vegetables; the citric acid of umeboshi helps in calcium absorption. The flavor of umeboshi is enhanced with olive oil or tahini as featured below.

UME DILL SALAD DRESSING

for 8 cups vegetables. Yield: ¾ cup

This dressing utilizes umeboshi plums and produces a thick dressing that tosses well with salad. At camp, this dressing is mixed with a salad of green leaf lettuce, red cabbage, sliced jicama, and garnished with blanched snow peas. The dinner menu includes azuki bean rice, corn on the cob, arame with carrots, dill pickle, and creamy celery soup, and is the *first meal* at camp. Cornellia Aihara designed this menu with festive colors of pink rice, black seaweed, yellow corn, green salad, and white soup, and it continues to be served in her honor as the introductory meal.

> **4 med umeboshi plums, whole**
> **¼ cup water**
> **½ small red onion, finely minced, ½ cup**
> **¼ cup olive oil**
> **2 Tbsp lemon juice**
> **1 tsp dried dill weed**

Simmer plums in water 5 to 10 minutes or until soft. Remove pits and purée plums in suribachi with the cooking liquid. Add minced onion and let sit 15 to 20 minutes. Add olive oil, lemon juice, and dill. Taste and adjust flavorings. Gently mix with salad.

TAHINI LEMON UME SALAD DRESSING

for 8 cups vegetables. Yield: ½ cup

This dressing is my favorite dressing for salads that include arugula and/or baby greens. At camp, the dressing is mixed with a salad of romaine lettuce, radish, red cabbage, carrot, and cucumber. The dinner menu includes polenta, pinto beans, long grain brown rice, corn on the cob, salad, dill pickle, corn chips, and cucumber salsa (recipe listed below under side dishes).

> **4 Tbsp tahini**
> **1 Tbsp umeboshi vinegar**
> **1 Tbsp lemon juice**
> **2 to 3 Tbsp water**

Cream tahini with umeboshi vinegar; add lemon juice and water in increments until thinned to desired consistency. Brands of tahini vary so adjust liquid content accordingly.

OLIVE OIL AND UMEBOSHI VINEGAR DRESSING

for 4 to 6 cups vegetables. Yield: ¼ cup

This dressing is delicious on many foods. I use it to dress salads or dab kale; one son douses brown rice; another son drowns pasta! A variation of this dressing is featured in the Brown Rice Salad, page 17.

3 Tbsp olive oil
1 Tbsp umeboshi vinegar

Mix ingredients together. Gently toss with salad or serve separately. To vary, add garlic pressed through a garlic press, dried mustard powder, dill weed, basil, or ground pepper. Allow to sit 10 to 15 minutes before using for best flavor. Shake well when serving.

Side Dishes

The following side dishes utilize cucumbers.

WAKAME ORANGE CUCUMBER SALAD

Yield: 2 ½ cups

This salad is a refreshing summer dish best made in small quantities and eaten fresh. At camp, it was featured in the menu plan in 2002 and 2003 and was prepared for lunch alongside Buckwheat Salad, page 18, kale, chickpeas, sautéed yellow squash, and miso soup.

1 six-inch piece of wakame, soaked in 1 cup water, will swell to
  2 Tbsp
Dressing
  1 tsp roasted sesame oil
  1 Tbsp brown rice vinegar
  1 Tbsp soy sauce
  2 Tbsp red onion, finely minced
  2 Tbsp minced celery
  1 cucumber, thin quarter rounds, 2 cups
  2 Tbsp parsley, finely chopped
  1 small orange, chopped, ¼ cup

Soak wakame 10 minutes. Drain. Separate leaves from stems. Chop leaves into ½-inch pieces. Reserve stems and soaking water for soup. Mix dressing. Fold wakame leaves and red onion in dressing and let stand 5 minutes; then mix with rest of ingredients.

Cucumber Relish

Yield: about 2 cups

This relish was inspired from one of Cornellia Aihara's quick pickle recipes she prepared at camp. It is served with the meal with fresh whole-wheat chapatis made in the bread baking class presented by Chuck Lowery of Pacific Bakery, Yeast Free. Also in this menu are humus, brown rice, green beans, and light vegetable soup.

> **1 cucumber, finely cut, 2 cups**
> **2 scallions, finely chopped, ½ cup**
> **¼ cup parsley, finely minced**
> **Dressing**
> > **1½ tsp toasted sesame oil**
> > **3 tsp soy sauce**
> > **1½ tsp ginger juice**
> > **1½ tsp lemon juice**

Cut all vegetables; mix dressing in bowl, add to vegetables and mix well. Taste and adjust seasonings if needed. Serve on lettuce leaves.

Cucumber Salsa

Yield: 4 cups

This salsa is served at camp with pinto beans, polenta, and salad with tahini lemon ume salad dressing (as above). This salsa is delicious, moist, and tomato-free! At camp, a tomato-based salsa is also available; however, the cucumber salsa usually disappears first.

> **1 large cucumber, chopped, 3 cups**
> **1 lime, juiced, 5 tsp**
> **1 red onion, minced, 1 cup**
> **1 stalk celery, finely minced, ¾ cup**
> **4 Tbsp finely minced cilantro**
> **4 Tbsp finely minced parsley**
> **1 Tbsp ume vinegar**

Combine all ingredients and let stand at least 1 hour before serving, stirring once or twice.

For additional condiment, dressing, and side dish recipes, see:
Avocado-Olive Spread—Annemarie Colbin, page 73.
Black Bean Salsa—Susanne Jensen, page 86.
Citrus-Flax Oil Vinaigrette—Meredith McCarty, page 95.
Dipping Sauce for Pot Stickers—Susanne Jensen, page 87.
Eggplant Appetizer—Annemarie Colbin, page 74.
Fermented Veggies—Packy Conway, page 78.
Flax Sunflower Basil Umeboshi Gomasio—Laura Stec, page 108.
Green Herb Coulis—Meredith McCarty, page 96.
Lemon-Miso Dressing or Sauce—Meredith McCarty, page 45.
Peanut-Apple-Miso Spread—Annemarie Colbin, page 75.
Quick Hors D'oeuvre: Avocado Sauerkraut Toast—Bob Carr, page 70.
Quick Summer Pickles—Bob Carr, page 71.
Salsa Verde Cruda (Fresh Green Salsa)—Dawn Pallavi, page 101.
Sesame Sauce—Susanne Jensen, page 88.
Shiitake Mushroom Sauce—Meredith McCarty, page 93.
Sweet Mustard-Garlic Vinaigrette—Meredith McCarty, page 95.
Tofu-Pickle Spread—Annemarie Colbin, page 74.
Wakame-Cucumber Salad—Ginat Rice, page 105.
White Bean Spread—Annemarie Colbin, page 73.

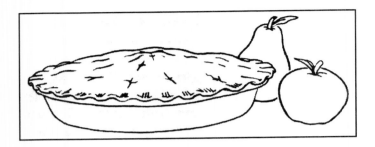

Favorite Desserts

Everyone loves dessert, whether at home or at camp. Camp provides challenges in preparing desserts, however, because there are no ovens for baking. All recipes are expanded 10 or more times and require care to make in quantity. The following recipes pass these criteria and please all campers.

COUSCOUS CAKE
Yield: 5 cups or 12 servings

> **1½ cups couscous**
> **4 cups apple juice**
> **¼ cup raisins**
> **¼ tsp sea salt**
> **pinch of cinnamon**
> **¼ cup almonds**
> **¼ tsp vanilla extract**

Place all ingredients, except vanilla extract, in a pot. If desired, almonds can be left out, roasted, and served as a garnish. Bring to a boil and simmer 10 minutes or until all liquid is absorbed and mixture is very thick. Stir in vanilla extract and remove from heat. Spoon into a dampened 8- by 10-inch cake pan and smooth top. Set until cool. Use sauce or topping as below, or serve with applesauce.

STRAWBERRY SAUCE FOR COUSCOUS CAKE
Yield: 2 cups or 12 servings

½ cup apple juice
1 pint strawberries, sliced, 2 cups
pinch of sea salt
3 to 4 tsp arrowroot powder

Bring apple juice to a boil. Add sea salt and strawberries. Bring to a boil again. Dilute arrowroot powder in 1 to 2 tablespoons juice and add to strawberries. Use the higher amount of arrowroot if berries are especially ripe and juicy. Stir constantly until thickened. Remove from heat. When cake is cool, cut into serving size pieces and spoon strawberry sauce on top.

GELLED STRAWBERRY TOPPING FOR COUSCOUS CAKE
Yield: 2 cups or 12 servings

This topping is used at French Meadows camp, since it is easier to serve in quantity than the strawberry sauce. Prepare topping and spoon on top of cake. When gelled, slice cake and serve.

1 pint strawberries, sliced, 2 cups
¼ cup apple juice
2 Tbsp agar flakes
¼ tsp sea salt

Bring all ingredients to a boil in an uncovered pot. Lower heat and simmer 5 minutes or until agar flakes are dissolved. Cool 5 minutes, then spread on top of prepared couscous cake. If cake is warm, it is okay. Allow to cool. When cake is cooled and the topping has gelled, slice and serve.

RICE PUDDING
Yield: 4½ cups or 5 to 6 servings

This recipe originated from *Natural Foods Cookbook* by Mary Estella, page 221. The altered recipe appears below.

3 cups cooked brown rice
2 cups apple juice

1 cup water
½ cup raisins
1 cinnamon stick
pinch of sea salt
½ tsp vanilla extract
1 tsp grated orange peel
½ cup walnuts, garnish
½ cup soymilk, garnish

Thoroughly mix and stir rice, juice, water, raisins, cinnamon, and sea salt in a heavy pot and bring to a boil. Simmer 30 minutes to soften rice. If rice absorbs all the liquid and starts to look dry, add more liquid, simmering up to an hour if needed. Once rice is very soft, add vanilla extract and orange peel and remove from heat. Serve with a garnish of toasted nuts and a splash of soymilk.

Peach Kanten
Yield: 7 cups or 8 servings

4 Tbsp agar flakes
4 cups apple juice
¼ tsp sea salt
4 to 6 peaches, pitted and sliced into crescents, 4 cups

Bring agar flakes, juice, and sea salt to a boil. Simmer over low heat with lid ajar until agar flakes are dissolved, from 5 to 10 minutes. Cool in pan 5 to 10 minutes. Place peaches in serving container. Ladle juice and agar mixture over peaches. Cool at room temperature until jelled, 1 to 1½ hours. If desired, refrigerate for faster jelling.

Almond (Peanut) Cereal Munchie
Yield: 16 to 24 servings

This recipe originated from *Be Nourished* by Rebecca Wood, page 72 (now available in *The Dakini Diet* from *www.rwood.com*). Camp needs required a few changes from the original recipe, as noted in parenthesis.

¼ cup almond butter (peanut butter)
⅓ cup rice syrup

½ cup chopped, roasted almonds
½ cup currants (raisins)
1 tsp lemon juice
½ tsp vanilla extract
½ tsp cinnamon or cardamom
¼ tsp sea salt
4 cups puffed millet (puffed rice)

Combine all but the puffed millet in a large bowl and stir to blend well. Add puffed millet and gently stir until well mixed. With moistened hands, press evenly into a lightly oiled 8½-inch baking pan. Let sit for 1 hour. Cut into 24 pieces.

Variations: Substitute peanuts and peanut butter for the almonds and almond butter. Substitute crispy rice or other cold breakfast cereal for the puffed millet.

For additional dessert recipes, see:

Almond Delight Cookies—Packy Conway, page 80.

Applesauce Pudding—Lisa Valantine, page 111.

Cantaloupe Pudding—David and Cynthia Briscoe, page 68.

Fresh Peach Compote with Almond-Orange Syrup—Meredith McCarty, page 93.

Kuzu Compote: Simplest, Quickest Dessert in the World—Bob Carr, page 71.

Lemon Tahini Crunch Cookies—Meredith McCarty, page 92.

Macrobiotic Halvah—Bob Carr, page 71.

Stovetop Mochi Pear Melt—David and Cynthia Briscoe, page 68.

Strawberry Couscous Cake—Lisa Valantine, page 110.

Twelve-Layer French Meadows Cake—Rebecca Wood, page 121.

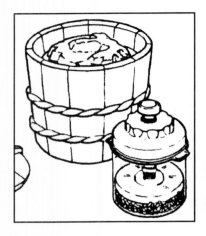

Umeboshi-Based Condiments

The condiments in this chapter are unique to this book—they are brought to camp but not prepared at camp. I designed these recipes for camp with the intention of introducing umeboshi and shiso to campers, and to provide condiments other than gomasio that are tasty, nutritious, and easy to prepare. Everyone loves them and asks for the recipes whenever they appear at meals.

The first five recipes feature umeboshi or shiso. Umeboshi has long been prized for its health-restorative qualities in Japanese and Macrobiotic cuisines. It is reputed to strengthen the digestive tract. Often it is used in teas or added to rice balls or norimake sushi. Shiso is the leaf of the reddish beefsteak plant, high in iron, and is pickled with umeboshi to give it a pink color.

I purchase umeboshi plums and shiso from Kazuko Yamazaki. Kazuko and her late husband, Junsei, are students of George Ohsawa and are pioneers in the Macrobiotic Movement, having devoted their lives to food production since the 1960s. Junsei worked on the first rice cake machines at Chico-san, in Chico, California, and developed Yinnies brand rice syrup, aka brown rice syrup. Together they established an orchard of Japanese plums and began the labor-intensive practice of producing traditional umeboshi. Plums are picked in the spring, dried in the sun, turned every day and night for a few weeks, and then fermented in a brine of salt and shiso leaves. Kazuko repeats the process each spring and summer and matures the plums for at least a year before selling them. (Plums available at camp and/or from Gold Mine Natural Foods.) She packages the plums with a little shiso on top.

For camp, I buy enough shiso leaves from Kazuko to make these recipes in quantity. To make these condiments at home, use the shiso that is packed with umeboshi or prepackaged shiso powder. Take special care to roast items separately from each other, and if you use the shiso packed with the umeboshi, air dry it thoroughly first. Shiso leaves reduce by one-fourth; e.g., 4 tablespoons shiso leaves will yield 1 tablespoon shiso powder.

SESAME SHISO

large amount—2¾ cups
  2 cups sesame seeds
  ¼ cup shiso powder or 1 cup shiso leaves

small amount—5 Tbsp
  4 Tbsp sesame seeds
  1½ tsp shiso powder or
  2 Tbsp shiso leaves

Wash and drain seeds. Roast. Process in food processor, or blender for the small amount, until all the seeds are crushed. Remove. If using dry shiso leaves, process shiso to a powder, using food processor for the large amount, coffee grinder for the small amount. Remove. Mix shiso powder and ground sesame together.

SUNFLOWER DULSE SHISO

large amount—3½ cups
  2 cups sunflower seeds
  2 cups dulse
  ¼ cup shiso powder or 1 cup shiso leaves
small amount—¾ cup
  ½ cup sunflower seeds
  ½ cup dulse
  1 Tbsp shiso powder or ¼ cup shiso leaves

Roast sunflower seeds and dulse in a 350 degree oven. Place on separate baking sheets. Spread seeds in a thin layer; flatten and separate dulse leaves as much as possible into a single layer. Roast until fragrant, sunflower seeds from 5 to 7 minutes, dulse about 5 minutes. If using shiso leaves process shiso to a powder in food processor for the large amount, coffee grinder or blender for the small amount. Remove. Process dulse and sunflower seeds together until seeds are crushed; then add shiso and mix together.

Ume Sesame

large amount—about 3 cups
   2 cups sesame seeds
   8 med umeboshi plums, pitted

small amount—⅓ cup
   ¼ cup sesame seeds
   1 med umeboshi plum, pitted

Roast seeds. Process until all seeds are crushed, using a food processor for large amount, blender for small amount. Add pitted umeboshi and process until well mixed. (Note that seeds must be thoroughly crushed before adding umeboshi.) If umeboshi paste is available, it can be substituted using 1 teaspoon paste per 1 umeboshi plum.

Shiso and Flax

Grind flax seeds (no need to roast) in a coffee grinder, for the best results. Remove. If using shiso leaves grind in coffee grinder, or blender if processing more than 4 tablespoons at a time. Mix ground flax and shiso powder together in equal proportions. For freshness, grind only enough flax to use within a week. (Note, shiso should be thoroughly dried before processing in a coffee grinder.)

Ume Walnut Ginger (moist condiment)

large amount—2¾ cups
   2 cups walnuts
   8 small umeboshi plums, pitted
   4 to 6 teaspoons ginger juice, freshly made
   1½ to 2 Tbsp water for thinning

> **small amount—5 Tbsp**
> **¼ cup walnuts**
> **1 small umeboshi plum, pitted**
> **½ to ¾ teaspoon ginger juice, freshly made**
> **about 1 teaspoon water for thinning**

Roast walnuts. Process in food processor, or blender for small amount, until all nuts are crushed. Add umeboshi and process. Add ginger juice and water to thin to desired consistency. Use within 3 to 4 days.

WAKAME ALMOND FISH

> **large amount—2¾ cups**
> **2 cups almonds**
> **16 small dried whole fish (2 Tbsp powder)**
> **36 inches wakame (3 Tbsp powder)**
>
> **small amount—about ¾ cup**
> **½ cup almonds**
> **4 small dried whole fish (1½ tsp powder)**
> **9 inches wakame (2¼ tsp powder)**

Whole dried fish are available in Japanese or Chinese food stores. They may be labeled Chuba Iriko, or Dried Sardines. They are used whole and provide a lot of calcium. Wakame also provides a lot of calcium. This condiment provides a lot of nutrition, and due to the almonds, a pleasant flavor.

Roast all items in a 350 degree oven until fragrant. Place on separate baking sheets. Roast almonds about 15 minutes, fish about 10 minutes, and wakame about 10 minutes.

While still warm, process in a food processor, one item at a time, and then remove. Wakame first; grind to as fine a powder as possible (36 inches will yield approximately 3 tablespoons powder as listed above). Fish second; grind to as a fine a powder as possible. Almonds third; process until all nuts are crushed; then add back to food processor with the wakame and fish and process together.

Cooking Class Recipes

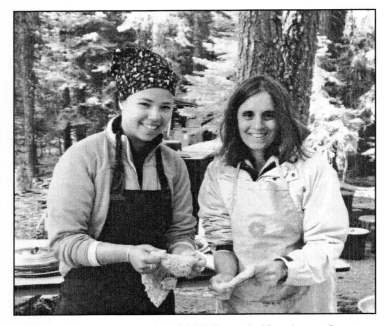

Flavia and Julia at the 2007 French Meadows Camp

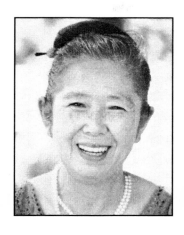

Recipes from
Cornellia Aihara

Cornellia Aihara was very resourceful and wasted nothing, using daikon greens and the white part of watermelon rinds. Her recipe for Green Pepper Watermelon Rind Oily Miso is legendary. The recipes provided here are an edited version of those published in the November/ December 1991 issue of Macrobiotics Today *and provide a sampling of Cornellia's camp cooking. Special thanks to Paul Sayre, Cornellia's assistant at the time, for compiling the recipes and adapting the portions to serve a family of four. – J.F.*

BROWN RICE WITH DAIKON GREENS

3 cups short grain brown rice
4 cups water
½ tsp sea salt
1 cup fresh daikon greens, finely chopped

Wash rice and place in a pressure cooker with water and ¼ tsp salt. Bring cooker up to pressure and cook for 45 minutes on a low heat using a heat diffuser. Remove the pressure cooker from the stove and allow pressure to come down slowly. Remove rice to a serving dish. Meanwhile, mix daikon greens with ¼ teaspoon salt and rub until green color comes out. Squeeze out green juice and discard. Mix daikon greens with the rice. They will "cook" in the hot rice.

KABOCHA POTAGE

> **1-2 tsp sesame oil**
> **1 medium onion, minced**
> **1 tsp sea salt**
> **1 stalk celery, diced**
> **¼ medium kabocha squash, cut into ¼-inch sections**
> **3 cups boiling water**
> **¼ cup rice cream powder or brown rice flour**
> **soy sauce to taste**

In a soup pot, heat oil, add onions, and sprinkle on ¼ teaspoon salt. Place otoshibuta (wooden cover) on onions and set heat on low. Cook onions until transparent, 5 to 10 minutes. Add celery and chopped kabocha and sprinkle on remaining salt. Let vegetables cook in own juices over medium-low heat for 15 minutes. Then add 2 cups boiling water and bring to a boil. Simmer for 10 minutes. Mix rice cream powder with 1 cup boiling water, add to vegetables, and cook for 20 minutes. Add soy sauce to taste and cook 10 minutes before serving.

KASHA (ROASTED BUCKWHEAT) WITH CURRY SAUCE

> **2 cups buckwheat**
> **4 cups boiling water**
> **½ tsp sea salt**
> **Curry Sauce**
> **1 ear fresh corn, remove kernels from cob and slice cob**
> **into 2 to 3 pieces**
> **3 cups boiling water**
> **3 tsp sesame oil**
> **¼-1 tsp curry powder**
> **¾ cup whole wheat pastry flour**
> **2 medium onions, minced**
> **1 Tbsp sea salt**
> **½ cup string beans, cut in ¼-inch pieces**
> **soy sauce to taste**

In a heavy pot, roast buckwheat until fragrant. Add boiling water, salt, and return to boil. Cover and simmer on low heat for 30 minutes.

Place corncob pieces in boiling water and cook on a low boil for 20 minutes. Remove cobs and save liquid for curry sauce.

In a heavy skillet, heat 2 teaspoons oil, add curry powder, and sauté briefly until fragrant. Add flour and sauté until flour is a rich yellow color, moving flour constantly to prevent burning. Remove from heat and cool.

In a heavy pot, heat the remaining oil, add onions, and ½ teaspoon salt. Sauté onions until brown. Add the green beans and cook for 3 to 5 minutes until the color of the green beans changes. Add corn and 1 cup of the corn cooking water. Bring to a boil. Add remaining salt and simmer until vegetables are tender. Stir 2 cups cool corn cooking water into the curry mixture, and then add to vegetables. Cook for 10 minutes. Add soy sauce to taste. Serve over Kasha.

GREEN PEPPER WATERMELON RIND OILY MISO

> 4 tsp sesame oil
> 2 cups watermelon rind, remove skin, cut white part into ¼-x-2-inch pieces
> ¼ tsp sea salt
> 1 medium green pepper, cut in ¼-inch slices
> 1-2 Tbsp barley miso

In a heavy pot, heat oil, add watermelon rinds, and sprinkle with salt. Cook for 10 minutes uncovered on medium heat until rinds are tender, stirring often. If water remains, cook on high heat to evaporate excess moisture. Add green peppers on top of watermelon rinds and simmer until peppers become bright green. Spread miso on top of rinds and peppers and cover. Simmer for 3 to 5 minutes to soften miso. Remove cover and stir until miso is fragrant. Serve.

COOKED LETTUCE SALAD

> ½ head Romaine lettuce
> 3 cups boiling water
> 1/3 tsp sea salt

Break the core from the lettuce and separate leaves. In a regular pot, add lettuce leaves to salted boiling water, and return to boil. When both sides of the leaves become bright green, remove from water and let leaves drain flat on a colander until cool. Squeeze out remaining water and cut in bite-size pieces. Serve with the following dressing.

Dressing
2 tsp lemon juice
1-2 tsp soy sauce
½ tsp ginger juice

Combine ingredients, then add more of each ingredient to taste.

CORN PUDDING
1/3 cup apples, cut in ½-inch slices
1/3 cup currants
3½ cups cold water
½ tsp sea salt
1 cup cornmeal
1 tsp cinnamon

Add sliced apples and currants to water. Bring to boil and add salt. Cover and cook for 20-30 minutes. Roast cornmeal in a heavy pot until fragrant. Sprinkle cornmeal 1 teaspoon at a time over cooking fruit and mix to avoid lumps. Return to boil, place heat diffuser under pot and cook on low boil covered for 45 minutes. Sprinkle on cinnamon and remove from stove and let cool. After 15 minutes stir and remove to a shallow pan. When completely cool, turn upside down, slice with a wet knife, and serve.

Cornellia Aihara (1926-2006) cofounded the George Ohsawa Macrobiotic Foundation and the Vega Study Center with her husband Herman. They also helped George Ohsawa establish the summer-camp tradition in 1960. Cornellia was the head cook at 38 consecutive camps in the United States and worked tirelessly to spread macrobiotics around the world. Her books include The Calendar Cookbook, The Do of Cooking, The Chico-San Cookbook *(also called* Macrobiotic Kitchen*), and* Natural Healing from Head to Toe.

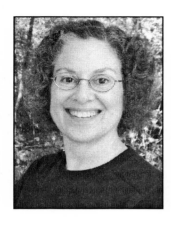

Recipes from
Lenore Baum

CHICKPEA STEW
8 servings

This soup quickly became a student favorite at my cooking school. It is so substantial that you can use it as a sauce over rice or noodles. Serve with steamed green vegetables to complete the meal. Pressure-cooking chickpeas saves a lot of time.

> ¾ **cup dried chickpeas**
> **2 cups water**
> **1, 6-inch strip kombu**
> ¼ **tsp unrefined sesame or olive oil**
> **2 medium onions, diced**
> **4 celery stalks, diced**
> **2 Tbsp shoyu**
> **2 Tbsp tahini**
> **1 cup butternut squash, diced**
> **1 tsp unrefined sea salt**
> **1 Tbsp fresh parsley, minced, to garnish**

The day before, pick over the chickpeas to remove debris and broken beans. Wash the beans and place them in a large bowl. Cover them with water, 2 inches above the level of beans and soak overnight.

Bring 2 cups of water to a boil in a pressure cooker. Add the rinsed chickpeas and return to a boil. Simmer uncovered for 5 minutes, skimming off foam that comes to the surface.

Meanwhile, cover the kombu with water and let soak for 5 minutes.

Cut it into ½-inch squares and add it to the pressure cooker. Lock the lid in place. Bring up to full pressure over high heat. Place a heat diffuser under the pressure cooker and reduce the heat. Maintain high pressure for 25 minutes.

Meanwhile, heat the oil in a nonstick skillet. Sauté the onions until slightly brown, about 15 minutes. Move the onions to one side of the pan and add a few more drops of oil to the cleared space. Sauté the celery for 1 minute. Whisk together shoyu and tahini in a small bowl and set aside.

Quick-release the pressure. Add the onions, celery, and squash. If the beans are not tender simmer until they are. Then add the salt and the tahini-shoyu mixture. Close the lid and let stand for 5 minutes, off the heat. Serve garnished with parsley.

Red Lentil Corn Chowder
10 servings

For years, this has been the favorite soup of my beginning students. Most tell me that even their meat-and-potato eaters love it!

6 cups water
1 cup red lentils
2 ears of corn, husked
1, 6-inch strip kombu
½ tsp unrefined sesame or olive oil
1 medium onion, diced small
2 carrots, cut into rounds, ¼-inch thick
3 celery stalks, diced small
3 Tbsp sweet, white miso
1 Tbsp fresh parsley, mined, to garnish, optional

Bring 6 cups of water to a boil in a large stock pot. Meanwhile, pick over the lentils to remove debris and set aside.

Add the corn to the stock pot and boil for 10 minutes. This makes a simple, sweet soup stock. Remove the cobs and allow to cool. Cut the kernels off the cobs and set aside. Discard the cobs. Add the rinsed lentils to the pot. Simmer uncovered for 15 minutes, skimming off foam from the surface until it subsides.

Meanwhile, cover the kombu with water and let soak for 5 minutes.

Cut it into ½-inch squares and add it to the pot.

Heat the oil in a large, nonstick skillet. Sauté the onion until translucent, about 5 minutes. Move the onion to one side of the skillet and add a few more drops of oil to the cleared space. Add the carrots and sauté for several minutes. Repeat with the celery. Add all the vegetables to the sock pot.

Place a heat diffuser under the pot. Simmer, with the lid ajar, until the lentils are soft and creamy, about 45 minutes. Stir occasionally.

Place a small amount of the hot chowder in a small bowl, add the miso, whisk until smooth and return it to the pot. Stir and serve garnished with parsley.

Variation: Substitute sweet, white miso for the chickpea miso.

Lenore Baum has lectured and taught at French Meadows camp many years. She is a Kushi Institute graduate with over 30 years experience and is the author of two books, Lenore's Natural Cuisine *and* Sublime Soups. *Lenore has a cooking school in Asheville, North Carolina. In addition to many classes on cooking and kitchen organizing, she maintains a list of superior cooking tools. Visit her website at* www. lenoresnatural.com.

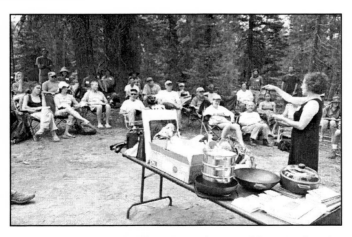

**Lenore demonstrating superior cooking tools at
the 2003 French Meadows Camp**

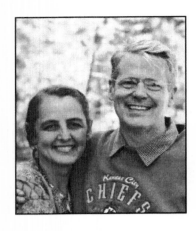

Recipes from

David and
Cynthia Briscoe

Soba Summer Salad

> 1½-inch bundle of soba noodles, broken into 2-inch long pieces
> boiling water to cook soba noodles
> 5 shiitake mushrooms, soaked until completely soft, reserve the
>   soaking water
> 1 Tbsp toasted sesame oil
> sea salt
> 6 inches of English cucumber, cut into thin diagonal
>   matchsticks
> 5 scallions, cut into ½-inch rounds
> 2 Tbsp toasted sesame seeds, coarsely chopped
> shoyu to taste

Preparing the soba noodles: Add broken soba noodles to rapidly boiling water. Stir. Shock twice using the following method: When the water starts to boil rapidly, add 2 cups of cold water. This method cools down the outside of the noodle, so it cooks evenly. The noodles are done when a piece of noodle is broken in two and it is a consistent color all the way through. However, do not overcook.

As soon as the noodles are cooked, drain them and rinse under cold water to stop the cooking. Drain once again.

Cooking the shiitake mushrooms: Slice the soaked shiitake into thin slices. Warm the oil in a skillet and sauté the shiitake, seasoning with a few small pinches of salt. Sauté until golden. Add enough shiitake soaking water to cover the mushrooms. Cover with a wet otoshibuta and a pot lid. Simmer over a low flame for 10 to 15 minutes. Reduce any remaining liquid.

Preparing the cucumbers: Sprinkle the cucumbers with a small amount of sea salt. Let them sit for 10 to 20 minutes and then squeeze off extra juice from the cucumbers.

Putting the salad together: Toss soba with the shiitake, cucumber, scallion, and sesame seeds. Season to taste with soy sauce. Serve immediately.

CARROT TOFU ASPIC

    1 lb block of tofu
    1½ cup water
    juice of 1 lemon (about 3 Tbsp)
    3 level Tbsp white miso
    3 rounded Tbsp agar flakes
    4 cups carrots cut in ½ rounds (about 7 carrots)
    ½ tsp sea salt
    3 or 4 stems parsley

Preparing the tofu: Rinse the tofu. Cut into ½-inch cubes. Place in a skillet arranged in one layer. Add ½ cup water, the lemon juice, and add the miso in dollops on top. Cover with a lid and cook over low heat with a heat diffuser under the pot. As the miso softens, spread it over the top of the tofu. Cook for 5 minutes more. Remove the lid and cook another 5 minutes to reduce the liquid by half.

Making the aspic: Place the agar flakes and ½ cup of water in a saucepan and soak for 10 to 15 minutes. Place on the stove and slowly bring to a simmer. Make sure the heat is very low. Continue simmering about 20 minutes with the lid slightly ajar on the pot, or until the agar is dissolved. Place the carrots, ½ cup water and ½ teaspoon salt in a pot and bring to a boil. Simmer the carrots over low flame, covered until soft. Drain liquid from carrots and add to the agar mixture.

Purée carrots in a Foley food mill or a blender. Mix the agar and carrots together and cook slowly another 5 minutes. Remove the pot from the stove and mix in the prepared tofu. Pour into an 8-inch square dish or a 9-inch round cake pan. Allow to cool and set up. Cut into squares or triangles. Garnish each slice with a sprig of parsley.

Cantaloupe Pudding

> **2 medium size ripe cantaloupes (about 14 cups diced,**
>   **6-7 lbs melon)**
> **¼ tsp sea salt**
> **1 cup unfiltered apple juice**
> **½ cup kuzu chunks**
> **1 Tbsp vanilla extract**
> **1 cup roasted cashew pieces for garnish**

Wash cantaloupes. Peel, cut in half and remove seeds. Slice into 1½-inch wedges and then dice. Place in a pressure cooker with salt and ½ cup apple juice. Bring to pressure. Cook 3 to 5 minutes.

Place pressure cooker in the sink and run cold water over the pressure cooker to bring down pressure quickly. Open lid of pressure cooker and mash with a potato masher. Return to stove to simmer.

Dissolve the kuzu in the remaining ½ cup of apple juice. Slowly add the kuzu mixture to the cantaloupe in a trickle. Whisk as you add the kuzu to prevent lumps. Cook until the kuzu turns clear. Turn off heat. Stir in vanilla.

Ladle into dessert cups and cool. Garnish with roasted cashew pieces just before serving.

Stovetop Mochi Pear Melt

> **5 bosc pears, sliced into ⅛-inch slices (about 6 cups sliced)**
> **½ cup unfiltered apple juice**
> **pinch of sea salt**
> **1 package cinnamon raisin mochi**

Place sliced pears in the bottom of a LeCreuset pot or a cast iron skillet. Add the apple juice and sprinkle with a pinch of salt. Mix. Cover the pot with a lid and simmer the pears until soft.

Slice the package of mochi into quarters and then slice each quarter block of mochi into two slices half the thickness. Remove the lid from the pot and lay the pieces of mochi on top of the pears. Return the lid to the pot and cook covered over low heat until the mochi melts.

If more than ¼ inch of apple juice remains in the bottom of the pot, remove lid and cook down apple juice. Serve while it is still warm.

Options: Mix about ¼ teaspoon cinnamon into pears. Add ¼ cup of raisins to the pears. Garnish with coarsely chopped roasted almonds.

STEAMED KABOCHA SALAD

> ½ medium kabocha squash (substitute 1 medium butternut squash if kabocha is unavailable), cut into chunks
> ½ medium red onion, cut into thin crescents
> 5 red radishes, cut into thin rounds
> 2 tsp umeboshi vinegar
> Dressing: Mix the following together
> 1 rounded Tbsp white miso
> 1 Tbsp sesame oil
> 1 to 2 Tbsp rice vinegar

Place the squash pieces in a steamer and steam for 5 minutes or until the squash can easily be pierced with a bamboo skewer. It should be tender, but still firm. Allow to cool completely and then place in a large bowl.

Mix the red onion, radishes and umeboshi vinegar. Place the red onion and radish mixture on top of the squash. Pour the dressing mixture on top next. Toss by flipping ingredients in the bowl or gently mix, taking care not to over mix and break up the squash pieces.

Serve immediately.

David and Cynthia Briscoe presented the first cooking classes at French Meadows camp, paving the way for many other teachers to follow. Over the years they have returned and delighted campers with original recipes. David and Cynthia worked at Vega Study Center with Herman and Cornellia Aihara and continue to provide macrobiotic education and seminars in Oroville, California, and wherever they travel. They host an active educational website and offer internet courses; audio, video, and CDs for home learning; certified counselor and cooking teacher career programs; and excellent personal macrobiotic guidance by phone (toll-free 877-622-2637 or 530-532-1918), in person, and online (www.macroamerica.com). David is coauthor of A Personal Peace.

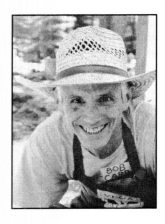

Recipes from
Bob Carr

Parsnip Delight

    2 to 3 parsnips, cubed
    water
    2 to 3 onions, sliced
    safflower, olive, or coconut oil
    2 Tbsp tahini
    1½ Tbsp brown rice vinegar
    ¼ to ½ tsp sea salt
    ¼ cup finely cut fresh parsley or 1½ Tbsp dried parsley flakes
    1 cup sweet brown rice flour

Place parsnips in pan with water to cover. Bring to a boil and simmer for twenty minutes or until tender, adding water as it boils away. Meanwhile, in a large frying pan, sauté onions in oil till clear, then add water to cover and simmer. Add tahini, brown rice vinegar, the cooked parsnips and cooking liquid, sea salt, and parsley. Then sprinkle sweet brown rice flour over all ingredients and mix. Stir gently until cooking liquid thickens, about 3 minutes.

Quick Hors D'oeuvre: Avocado Sauerkraut Toast

    tahini
    sauerkraut
    avocado
    100% sour dough rye bread

Toast bread (any bread will do, if sour dough rye is unavailable). Spread a thin layer of tahini evenly on surface of toast. Crush about ¼ meat from avocado with tines of fork and spread on toast with tahini spread. Cover with thin layer of sauerkraut. Cut toast 3 x 3 to make 9 servings.

Quick Summer Pickles

Pour shoyu into a glass peanut butter size jar until ¼ full, add an equal amount of brown rice vinegar (Genmai Su). Submerge slices of onion, Chinese cabbage, and any other veggies you want. Let set at least an hour, rinse and serve. The finer you slice the veggies, the quicker they pickle. If you want to make the pickles and serve them a day or more later, use bigger slices. It's that simple.

Kuzu Compote: Simplest, Quickest Dessert in the World

2 cups pitted prunes (or dried apples, peaches, or other fruit)
1½ tablespoons kuzu
1 cup of cold water

Place pitted prunes (or dried apples, peaches, or other fruit) in a sauce pan and cover with water. Bring to a boil, then simmer until fruit is completely softened—about 6 to 8 minutes. Meanwhile, dilute kuzu in a cup of cold water and stir until completely dissolved. Bring heat under softened fruit back up to high and add diluted kuzu and water, stirring constantly. When the milky kuzu mixture starts to thicken, boil and turn translucent, simmer for one minute more, stirring continually. Serve hot in winter or let cool for summer. This can also be used as a topping for muffins, couscous cake, or a spread for toast.

Macro Halvah

1 cup whole wheat flour (roasted until golden)
1 cup tahini
3 Tbsp maple syrup
½ tsp vanilla extract
3-4 pinches sea salt
10 roasted almonds

Roast one cup fresh ground whole wheat flour until golden (not quite brown, definitely not dark brown). It's okay if you don't have fresh ground flour, use organic whole wheat bread flour.

Mix tahini, maple syrup, and vanilla. Mix whole wheat flour and sea salt. Combine and press into flat cookie sheet. Cut into squares and push a roasted almond into each halvah square.

QUICK-AND-EASY TANGY COLE SLAW

½ head cabbage
¼ tsp sea salt
1 to 2 small carrots
1½ to 2 Tbsp Vegenaise or Nasoya salad dressing
   (creamy dill)
1 small lemon, juiced

Grate cabbage, sprinkle with sea salt, then mix and squeeze cabbage by hand. Grate carrots and mix with cabbage. Mix Vegenaise or Nasoya salad dressing and juice from lemon. Let set for 10 minutes, preferable in refrigerator if hot weather.

Bob Carr has over 35 years of macrobiotic teaching and counseling experience. He founded the East West Center of Cleveland, as well as the Cleveland Tofu Company. Author of The Energy of Food—sorry, only currently available in the Czech language—and editor of the Macro News Letter, Bob has taught macrobiotics throughout Europe, Asia, Australia, Canada and of course the USA. He was a director of the Kushi Institute of Germany, as well as having taught at the KI in Becket and Japan. Along with lecturing and counseling at French Meadows, he highly enjoyed being head cook one year and didn't burn the beans or set the woods on fire. He is currently researching Parkinson's disease from all angles—a very macro approach.

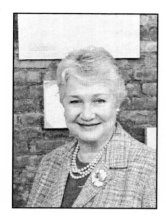

Recipes from

Annemarie Colbin

from The Book of Whole Meals

Avocado-Olive Spread

Serves: 4
Time: 10 minutes

> **1 ripe avocado**
> **2 Tbsp lemon juice**
> **6 black Greek olives**
> **sea salt to taste**
> **radishes, sliced**

Scoop the avocado pulp into a bowl; add the lemon juice and mash with a fork. Pit and finely chop the olives; stir into the avocado. Add salt to taste. Garnish with sliced radishes and serve with whole grain toast or crackers.

White Bean Spread

Serves: 4
Time: 5 minutes

> **Leftover white bean vinaigrette, leftover (page 75)**
> **3 to 4 Tbsp water**
> **shoyu (natural soy sauce) to taste**
> **parsley**

Using a fork, mash the beans thoroughly in a mixing bowl. Moisten with the water and continue mashing until smooth. Add shoyu to taste. Garnish with parsley and serve with whole grain toast or crackers.

EGGPLANT APPETIZER

Serves: 4
Time: 15 minutes, 30 hours; 15 minutes, 30 minutes

> **1 medium-sized eggplant**
> **sea salt**
> **½ tsp oregano**
> **½ tsp basil**
> **2 to 3 cups water**
> **2 Tbsp lemon juice**
> **2 Tbsp olive oil**

Wash the eggplant and cut into ½-inch round slices. Sprinkle each slice liberally with salt and stack in a crock or bowl. Place a plate on top of the slices with stones or other weights on top of the plate; allow to stand for at least 30 hours. Discard the water that has been extracted from the eggplant and cut the eggplant into bite-size chunks.

Combine the eggplant, oregano, and basil in a 2-quart pot with water to cover; simmer for 15 minutes. Drain the eggplant and allow to cool. Combine the lemon juice and olive oil; add to the eggplant and toss well. Allow to marinate for at least 30 minutes. The mixture will keep for 5 to 6 days in the refrigerator.

TOFU-PICKLE SPREAD

Serves: 4
Time: 10 minutes

> **1, 8-ounce cake tofu**
> **2 Tbsp unrefined sesame oil**
> **1 cucumber dill pickle**
> **1 Tbsp sesame salt (gomashio) or to taste**
> **sprouts**
> **1 red pepper**

Using a fork, mash the tofu in a bowl or suribachi; blend in the sesame oil. Chop the pickle very fine and add to the tofu, mixing well; add sesame salt to taste. Garnish with sprouts and strips of red pepper and serve with whole grain toast or crackers.

PEANUT-APPLE-MISO SPREAD

Serves: 4
Time: 5 minutes

> ½ cup peanut butter
> 4 Tbsp apple butter
> 1 to 2 Tbsp miso
> 3 Tbsp water
> peanuts, roasted

Combine the first 4 ingredients in a bowl, mixing with a wooden spoon until creamy. Garnish with roasted peanuts and serve with whole grain toast or crackers.

WHITE BEANS VINAIGRETTE

Serves: 4
Time: 10 minutes; 3 hours, 15 minutes

> 2 cups dry baby lima beans, soaked 6 to 8 hours in advance
> 8 cups water
> 1 small carrot
> 1 small onion
> 2 parsley sprigs
> 1 tsp sea salt
> 2 Tbsp chives
> ½ red bell pepper
> 1 handful parsley
> 2 whole scallions
> Vinaigrette: Combine the ingredients, mixing well with a fork
> 1 tsp umeboshi plum pate
> 4 Tbsp brown rice vinegar
> 2 Tbsp olive oil

Place the beans and water in a 3-quart pot and soak for 6 to 8 hours. Add the whole carrot and onion and the parsley sprigs to the beans; simmer for 1 hour. Add salt 10 minutes before removing beans from heat. Discard the carrot, onion, and parsley sprigs; drain the beans and cool to room temperature.

Chop the chives, red pepper, parsley, and scallions. In a 1-quart bowl, combine 3 cups cooked beans, chives, red pepper, parsley, and scallions. Toss with Vinaigrette and marinate for at least 15 minutes.

Annemarie Colbin, Ph.D., founder and CEO of the Natural Gourmet Institute for Health and Culinary Arts, New York City, New York. Telephone: 212-645-5170. Website: www.naturalgourmetschool.com. *See also Dr. Colbin's personal website,* www.foodandhealing.com, *and her video blog,* www.holisticanarchy.com.

Annemarie has authored three books: The Book of Whole Meals, The Natural Gourmet, *and* Food and Healing. *She attended camp in 1996 and has supported G.O.M.F. for many years. We are pleased to share these recipes from* The Book of Whole Meals.

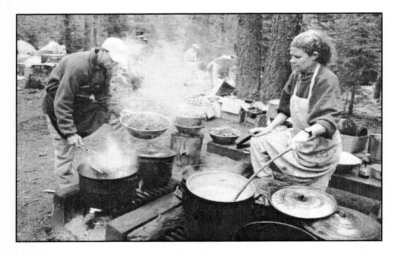

Morgan Jones and Saci McDonald Cooking at the 2005 French Meadows Camp

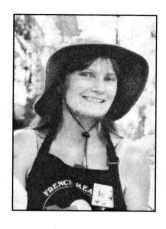

Recipes from

Packy Conway
and James Brunkow

James and Packy's Burdock Ribs

This was a favorite of our kids as they were growing up. Ian, our third son, scored 5 goals in soccer in one game and the coach asked, "What did you feed him this morning?" I told him Burdock Ribs! He replied, "Feed him that before every game." We use all organic ingredients.

6 burdock
1 small onion
2-3 Tbsp of olive oil
2 cloves of garlic
soy sauce to taste
1-2 Tbsp of chili powder

Cut burdock into very long diagonal pieces. Cut the onion into small diced pieces. Heat the oil for one minute in a cast iron saucepan. Add onion and sauté until translucent, then add the burdock. Sauté for 5 minutes together with the onion. Add garlic by squeezing through a garlic press. Sauté for another 5 minutes. Add soy sauce to taste and chili powder.

Continue sautéing the burdock on low heat until it is soft. I like mine well done, so I cook them longer. These are fun finger food and a scrumptious snack throughout the year.

FERMENTED VEGGIES

Use all organic ingredients—whatever is in season and cheap. This recipe can be made in a large Japanese press. All of our friends and family enjoy our fermented veggies. We serve them quite frequently.

> **1 large cabbage**
> **½ yellow onion (red works too)**
> **½-1 carrot**
> **½ cauliflower**
> **½-1 serrano pepper**
> **3 cloves of garlic**
> **2 tsp sea salt**

Cut the cabbage into quarters. Slice each quarter very fine. Cut the onion into halves and dice fine as well. Cut the carrot into very thin matchsticks. Cut the cauliflower into small pieces. Cut the pepper into very small pieces. (Be careful not to touch your eyes working with the pepper—wash hands after cutting it.)

Layer all ingredients into a Japanese press, starting first with some cabbage, then some carrot, onion, cauliflower, and garlic. Sprinkle some salt onto the first mixture. Continue with the layering and salt until all ingredients are in the press. Turn the handle at the top to press the veggies down. As liquid starts to cover the veggies, put more pressure on the layered mixture by turning the knob at the top of the press. This mixture should be kept in a dark cool place. Check it in about 8 to 10 days. It depends upon the weather how fast the pickling process will take.

PACKY'S MINESTRONE SOUP

This delicious soup is so filling during the fall/winter months. I found if I adjust the amount of beans and veggies, I can make it lighter for the spring/summer months as well. (Use organic ingredients.)

> **1 onion**
> **1 carrot**
> **½ burdock**
> **¼ cabbage**
> **3 stalks celery**
> **½ yam**
> **olive oil**

6 cups filtered water
6-inch piece wakame
1 cup garbanzos (already cooked)
½ cup lentils (uncooked)
spices to taste: pepper/salt/oregano
1 can of organic tomato sauce (optional)
1 cup peas (fresh or frozen)

Cut all veggies into bite-sized pieces (except peas). Sauté lightly in large soup pot for 5 minutes. Add water to the pot, then wakame. Let cook for about 20 minutes together. Add cooked garbanzos and add uncooked lentils at this time. Cook for about 50 minutes. Add spices and tomato sauce at this time. Let cook all day for hours. Right before serving, add the fresh or frozen peas for color. This soup is so delicious.

Variations: Cook organic noodles of choice. I prefer Tinkyada brown rice. The next day to use leftover soup, pour a ladle of soup over the noodles and enjoy. In warmer weather, add less beans and veggies and keep the same amount of broth.

PACKY'S RAW CRACKERS

These crackers are enzyme rich as they do not cook above 95 degrees in the dehydrator, which is necessary. They are super healthy and taste good too. They make good traveling food. I bring these down to French Meadows Summer Camp every year and share with my camper friends. They stay fresh all the way to camp, through camp (2 weeks) and for the return trip home.

1 cup sunflower seeds
½ cup flax seeds
1 tsp salt
½ Tbsp agave syrup

Soak all seeds for at least 8 hours. Drain off the liquid into a small bowl. The flax seeds will have a very gelatinous texture. Place seeds into a cuisinart. Ground the seeds up until you get a gloppy mixture. You may need to add a little of the poured off liquid. Add the salt and agave syrup.

Using a dehydrator—place the mixture onto the mylar sheets that go on the racks to the dehydrator. Spread the mixture out making a huge flat rectangle approximately ½-inch thick. Put the crackers into the dehydrator at 95 degrees to dry. After about 5 hours, make cuts into the mixture so that it is easier to cut when finally dried. (I cut across 3x each way like a tick-tack-toe board.) Flip mixture over to the other side after approximately 10 hours. Then continue to dehydrate for another 8 hours. These crackers are so tasty.

Variations: Try adding orange or lemon zest. Try adding chili powder and ume vinegar. Try adding a few soaked almonds and goji berries (wolfberries). Try using a small piece of banana and a little shredded coconut.

ALMOND DELIGHT COOKIES

Everyone loves these cookies (use organic ingredients).

> 1½ cups rolled oats (ground)
> 1 cup soft white wheat flour
> ¼ tsp baking soda
> ½ tsp salt
> 1 tsp cinnamon
> 1 cup chopped almonds fine
> ½ cup vegan choco chips (optional)
> ½ cup light oil
> ½ cup maple syrup or agave syrup
> 2 tsp vanilla or almond extract

Grind oats in a cuisinart. Add all dry ingredients together in a large bowl. Then mix together all wet ingredients in a smaller bowl. Combine the wet ingredients to the dry bowl. Try not to over mix the ingredients. Place spoonfuls of the mix onto a cookie sheet in ball shapes. Flatten the cookies using a fork dipped into water if needed. I usually get 20 cookies per sheet. Preheat oven to 350 degrees. Cook for 10 to 15 minutes until golden brown.

Variations: Add orange zest or ginger to this recipe. Use cashews instead of almonds. Add raisins or goji berries (wolfberries).

Packy Conway has attended camp, along with James Brunkow and their family, for almost every year since the late 1970s. She organized and conducted the Kid's Program for many years and now is one of the co-head cooks. James is the driving force in the kitchen, maintaining the fires and providing hot water for all uses. Packy and James are expert cooks: Packy excels at fermented vegetables and dried snacks and James at sourdough bread, organic beer, and kombucha tea. They live in Portland, Oregon.

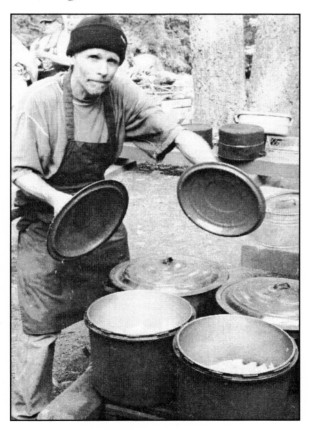

**James Cooking at the 2007 French
Meadows Camp**

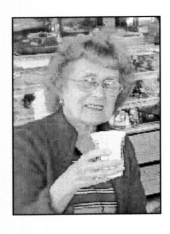

Recipes from

Yvette DeLangre

Stir-Fried Vegetables

    olive or sesame oil
    garlic (germ removed) finely chopped
    ginger root, chopped
    onion sliced from yin to yang in crescents
    celtic salt
    Nappa cabbage
    broccoli
    cauliflower
    carrots cut into match sticks
    soy sauce

Heat up oil in wok. Sauté garlic, add ginger and sauté until fragrant, add onions, sauté until transparent, add a little salt. (Salt will draw water out of the vegetables and they will cook in their own juice.) Add Nappa cabbage, broccoli, cauliflower, and last carrots. Add soy sauce to taste. Cover and cook about 5 minutes.

Never lift up the cover during cooking, if you do the greens will turn gray and will not taste good. If the lid is lifted accidently, finish cooking without a lid, stirring occasionally. If all the liquid is not evaporated you can thicken with arrowroot or kudzu.

We cook vegetables from yin to yang. Carrots being very yang are added last—they don't need to be yangized. Any combination of vegetables may be used.

Hiziki Side Dish

1 oz hiziki
water to cover
1 Tbsp sesame oil
a pinch of Celtic salt
2½ Tbsp soy sauce
leftover kombu, soaked (if dry) and cut into strips 2 inches
(optional)

Wash hiziki in cold water to remove sand. Soak for about 15 minutes. Save the soaking water. Cut hiziki in about 2 inches length. Heat oil in a deep sauce pan and sauté hiziki until it has a nice fragrance. Slowly add about 1 cup of water from soaking. Bring to a boil, add the salt, a little soy sauce and the kombu strips. Simmer for 45 minutes to one hour or longer. The longer the cooking the better the flavour.

Several times during the cooking and at the end add a little soy sauce. It should taste salty but not too salty.

Variations: Cut fresh lotus root or carrots into slivers, sauté in sesame oil, add hiziki, and continue cooking as above. You can also sprinkle with toasted sesame seed.

Rice Croquettes (Deep-Fried)

rice, cooked
oil
soy sauce

Shape sticky rice into cylinders and deep fry in safflower oil. Season with soy sauce.

Yvette DeLangre is a long-time teacher at French Meadows camp. Along with her late husband, Jacques, Yvette is a student of George Ohsawa and is well-versed in the healing strength of macrobiotics. Jacques and Yvette were instrumental in importing Celtic sea salt in the USA and established the Grain and Salt Society. See website at www. celticseasalt.com.

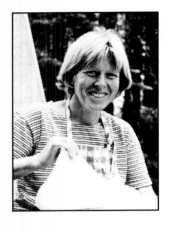

Recipes from

Susanne Jensen

ITALIAN WHITE BEAN HUMMUS

> **2 cups cooked white beans**
> **¼ cup tahini**
> **¼ cup lemon juice**
> **2 cloves garlic**
> **½ teaspoon cumin powder**
> **dash cayenne**
> **2 Tbsp olive oil**
> **¼-½ cup bean juice or water**

Combine beans, tahini, lemon juice, garlic, cumin, and cayenne in the food processor. Blend and gradually add oil and water until the mixture has a creamy consistency. Serve with warm pita bread triangles and chopped tomato.

SESAME SAUCE

> **¼ cup sesame tahini**
> **2 Tbsp apple cider vinegar**
> **juice of one orange**
> **1 clove garlic, minced**
> **¼ tsp sea salt**
> **dash of pepper**

Whisk all ingredients together in a small bowl.

GREENS WITH GRATED BEET AND ORANGE

1 Tbsp olive oil
1 onion, diced
1 bunch chard, sliced thin
1 bunch collard greens, sliced thin
½ tsp salt
1 beet, grated fine
2 oranges cut into small pieces

Heat oil in a wok and add onion. Sauté for 3-5 minutes. Add greens and salt and sauté until soft, 5-7 minutes. Transfer greens into a serving bowl and mix with beet, oranges, and dressing.

Dressing
¼ cup freshly squeezed orange juice
juice from half a lemon
1 tsp mustard
2 Tbsp olive oil
½ tsp salt

Whisk all ingredients together in a small bowl.

CARROT LIME SOUP

2 Tbsp oil
1-inch fresh ginger, minced
1 onion, chopped
7 medium carrots, chopped roughly
1 sweet potatoes, chopped into cubes
2 celery ribs, chopped
4 cups water
juice from 1 lime
1½ tsp salt
pepper, to taste
parsley for garnish, chopped

Sauté ginger, onions, carrot, sweet potato and celery for 2-3 minutes or until onion is tender. Add water and simmer for 20 minutes or until veggies are tender. Add lime juice, salt and pepper and purée in blender until smooth. Serve soup garnished with a little parsley.

Pinto Beans and Onions

1 cup pinto beans
4 cups water
2 large onions
2 cloves garlic (optional)
2 Tbsp olive oil
1 tsp sea salt, or to taste

Check beans for stones and dirt by sorting through a small amount at a time on a large plate. Rinse and soak for 6 to 8 hours.

Drain beans. Add fresh water just to cover, and bring to a boil. When boiling, skim off white foam gathering on top. Simmer beans for 1 hour. Add a little more water if needed.

Cut onions into half-moon slices. Peel and mince garlic. Place onion and garlic with oil and a pinch of salt in a pot and sauté until onion gets soft. Add beans and salt and simmer for 30 minutes.

Black Bean Salsa

2 cups chopped tomatoes
2 cups cooked black beans
1 cup diced red onion
1 large jalapeno, seeded and minced
½ cup loosely packed chopped cilantro
1 Tbsp chopped parsley
2 cloves garlic, chopped
1 tsp salt
juice of one lime or lemon
1 Tbsp olive oil
corn tortillas or crispy corn chips

Combine the first seven ingredients in a mixing bowl. Season with salt. Add the lime juice and olive oil. Mix well. Spoon into a serving bowl and serve with corn tortillas or corn chips.

Pot Stickers

Natalie Jung taught me this recipe.

Filling
4 scallions, cut very thin

3 cups bok choy, chopped fine
1 carrot, finely grated
⅓ pound tofu, crumbled
2 tsp grated ginger
½ tsp sea salt
1½ Tbsp soy sauce
2 tsp toasted sesame oil
Dough
  2 cups whole wheat pastry flour
  2 cups unbleached white flour
  1½ tsp sea salt
  2 Tbsp oil
  1 ¾ cup boiling water
For Cooking
  oil
  water

Mix vegetables, tofu, ginger, salt, soy sauce and sesame oil in a bowl.

To make dough, measure the 2 kinds of flour and pour into a bowl. Add salt, oil, and boiling water and mix well. When cool enough to handle knead until all flour has been worked into dough. Roll dough into a 9-inch long log about 1½ inch in diameter. Slice into ½-inch pieces and with a rolling pin roll each piece into thin circles.

Place a tablespoon of vegetable-tofu mixture in the center. Gather up sides to create a half moon shape and pinch the edges to seal pot stickers.

Heat 2 tablespoons of oil in a skillet. Place pot stickers in a skillet, close together, but not touching. Cook for about 3-4 minutes. Add ½ cup of water, cover skillet and steam for 5-7 minutes or until all the water is evaporated. Serve pot stickers with dipping sauce.

Dipping sauce
  ⅓ cup soy sauce
  1 Tbsp rice vinegar
  2 tsp ginger juice
  2 tsp water

Mix everything in a small bowl.

NAPPA CABBAGE QUINOA ROLLS WITH SESAME SAUCE

1 Tbsp olive oil
1 carrot, diced
1 cup finely chopped cabbage
1 stalk celery, finely diced
½ onion, finely diced
1 cup quinoa
2 tsp vegetable powder
2 cups boiling water
½ tsp sea salt
½ cup chopped parsley
½ cup toasted chopped sunflower seeds
8-10 Nappa cabbage leaves quickly cooked in a large
   pot of water

Heat olive oil and sauté carrot, cabbage, celery and onion for 2 minutes. Add quinoa, vegetable powder, boiling water and salt and bring to a boil. Reduce heat to low and simmer for 15-20 minutes or until all the water is gone. Add parsley and sunflower seeds and mix well.

Roll quinoa pilaf up inside cooked Nappa cabbage leaves. If needed use a tooth pick to hold it together. Serve with sesame sauce.

Susanne Jensen is a graduate of the Kushi Institute. She has taught cooking classes in her native Europe and the United States for more than 25 years. For the past 9 years Susanne has been an employee of Berkeley Unified School District. There she teaches middle school students how to cook with fruits, vegetables, grains and beans, as well as teaching them the health benefits of eating a vegetable-based diet. Susanne is currently co-head cook at French Meadows camp.

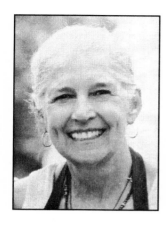

Recipes from
Barb Jurecki-Humphrey

TEMPEH MOCHI REUBEN SANDWICH

1 block tempeh
1-2 cloves garlic
olive oil to sauté
⅓ to ½ cup soy sauce
1 cup water
½ block plain mochi cut crosswise like French fries
⅛ cup nutritional yeast flakes
½ cup sauerkraut
6 slices rye bread
mustard, lettuce, pickle

Sauté tempeh in garlic and olive oil. Mix soy sauce in water and add to skillet. Lay strips of mochi across top of tempeh. Sprinkle nutritional yeast flakes. Cover and simmer until mochi is melted. Add sauerkraut. Cut into slabs and place on rye bread. Add mustard, lettuce, and dill pickle. Serve open face or as a sandwich.

BASIC CONGEE RECIPE

Congee is rice cooked with a lot of water, usually overnight, to produce a soft porridge that is healing, delicious, and satisfying. Barb has perfected the art of making congee and varies the ingredients put into her crock pot. Her cooklet, The Congee Cooklet, *has numerous recipes and suggestions for creating your own combinations. – J.F.*

Cook overnight
½ cup Job's tears (hato mugi)
8 cups water
¼ cup red lentils
1-inch piece kombu
1 pinch sea salt
¼ tsp garlic or garlic powder
¼ tsp cinnamon

To prepare congee, place all ingredients in a slow cooker in the evening and set on medium overnight. It makes a wonderful breakfast. In the morning add chopped scallions, kale, or other leafy greens. Season with miso, shoyu, maple syrup, or honey.

CAULIFLOWER CURRY COCONUT SOUP

½ tsp curry powder
1 Tbsp Virgin coconut oil
2 tsp olive oil
1 medium onion diced
¼-½ tsp white pepper
3 cups cut up cauliflower
2½ cups boiling water
¼-½ tsp sea salt
optional: can organic coconut milk
parsley garnish

In pressure cooker, sauté curry in coconut oil and olive oil. Add diced onion and white pepper. Sauté until translucent. (Optional: remove 2 tablespoons sautéed onion for garnish.) Add cauliflower and sauté 4 minutes while turning and coating. Add boiling water. (Adjust for thicker or thinner soup) Bring to pressure and cook under pressure 15 minutes. Add salt to taste. (Add and heat optional coconut milk) Garnish with parsley and optional onion garnish.

SPICY UDON SALAD

Recipe used with the kind permission of Eden Foods, Inc. of Clinton, Michigan. Their many excellent-quality foods are available at natural and health food stores and at www.edenfoods.com. *– J.F.*

> 1 cup arame or hiziki
> 1 cup water
> 2 medium carrots cut into matchsticks
> 1 package udon or soba noodles
> 3-4 green onions thinly sliced
> **Dressing**
> 1 Tbsp Eden hot pepper sesame oil
> 1 Tbsp Eden toasted sesame oil
> ¼ cup ume vinegar
> ¼ cup tahini
> 2-3 cloves garlic minced
> ⅛ cup water or stock

Soak arame or hiziki in water 10 minutes. Simmer for 10 to 15 minutes until water is absorbed. Lightly steam carrots. Rinse with cold water. Cook pasta as package directs. Mix pasta, arame and green onions. Prepare dressing. Add to salad. Mix well. Chill before serving optional.

Barb Jurecki-Humphrey has authored two books, The Congee Cooklet, *and* The Feng Shui for Harmony Handbook. *Barb has attended camp consecutively for many years, cooking in the kitchen, presenting classes on Feng Shui, and teaching cooking classes, both to adults and to children. She lives in Telluride, Colorado; e-mail:* jurecki@starband. net.

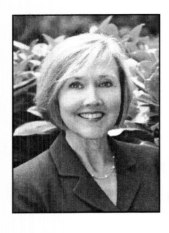

Recipes from

Meredith McCarty

LEMON TAHINI CRUNCH COOKIES

Lemon juice and zest add sparkle to this cookie made richer with sesame tahini. Makes 10 to 12.

- 1½ cups oatmeal
- ¾ cup whole wheat pastry flour
- ¾ cup unbleached white flour
- ½ cup sesame seeds, toasted
- 1 tsp aluminum-free baking powder
- ½ tsp sea salt
- ½ cup light vegetable oil
- ¼ cup sesame tahini
- ¾ cup brown rice syrup
- zest of half a lemon
- 2 Tbsp lemon juice
- 1 tsp vanilla

Preheat oven to 350 degrees. Line two baking sheets with parchment paper or brush with oil. In a medium-large bowl, mix dry ingredients. In a smaller bowl, whisk together wet ingredients. Stir into dry.

Transfer heaping tablespoons of dough to baking sheet, leaving two inches of space between cookies. If uniformity is important, use a ¼- or ⅓-cup scoop. Cookies will spread, but you may choose to flatten batter with the back of a fork to make 3- or 4-inch round shapes ½-inch thick. Dip scoop and/or fork in water to keep it from sticking.

Bake cookies until edges are golden, about 20 minutes.

FRESH PEACH COMPOTE WITH ALMOND-ORANGE SYRUP

Makes 6 servings or 4½ to 6 cups.

> **Almond-Orange Syrup**
> > ¼ tsp almond extract
> > ½ cup orange juice
> > ½ cup brown rice syrup
> > Zest of an orange
> > Zest of a quarter of a lemon
> > Few grains sea salt
> **Fruit and Garnishes**
> > 2 lbs peaches, 4 peaches or 6 cups, halved and cut in
> > > ½-inch slices, then in half crosswise
> > ¼ cup slivered almonds, toasted
> > fresh mint sprigs for garnish

In a bowl big enough to hold the peaches, whisk the syrup ingredients together. Add the peaches. You may serve this compote immediately or allow it to marinate. A lot of liquid comes out of the peaches as they sit—fruit is submerged in syrup after an hour—adding volume and a greater depth of flavor to the syrup. Gently stir occasionally with a rubber spatula.

Serve both fruit and syrup. Garnish with almonds and mint.

CUMIN-SCENTED QUINOA WITH SHIITAKE MUSHROOM SAUCE

Makes 3 to 4 servings or 3½ to 4 cups

> **Kombu-Shiitake Broth: Makes 2¾ cups**
> > 1 quart water
> > 3-inch piece kombu sea vegetable
> > 4 large fresh or dried shiitake mushrooms
> **Cumin-Scented Quinoa**
> > 1 cup quinoa
> > 1½ cups water
> > 1 tsp olive or sesame oil
> > 2 shallots, minced
> > 1 large clove garlic, minced
> > ¼ pound fresh shiitake mushrooms, 2 cups, stems trimmed,
> > > caps and stems diced small
> > 1 small carrot, diced small

¼ **tsp sea salt**
1½ **tsp natural soy sauce**
1 **bay leaf**
1 **tsp cumin powder**
¼ **cup pine nuts, lightly toasted (8 minutes at 300 degrees)**
¼ **cup parsley, finely chopped, and 4 leaves for garnish**
1 **carrot, thinly sliced, boiled 5 minutes, and cut with hors d'oeuvre cutters for garnish**
Shiitake Mushroom Sauce: Makes a little more than 1 cup
1 **cup** *Kombu-Shiitake Broth*
1½ **to 2 Tbsp natural soy sauce, start with less**
2½ **Tbsp kuzu root starch or arrowroot powder**
water

To prepare broth for sauce, bring ingredients to boil in a 2-quart saucepan. Turn heat down to simmer covered for 10 minutes. Strain out kombu and shiitake and reserve for another use.

In a bowl, generously cover grains with cool water. Swish them with your hand to release any dirt. Drain, add measured amount of water, and allow to soak for an hour. Drain, and measure water that remains before discarding it.

In a 2-quart saucepan, heat the oil with 2 tablespoons water. Add the shallots, garlic, mushrooms, carrot, and salt. Sauté the vegetables for 2 to 3 minutes. Add the same amount of fresh water as the amount you discarded from soaking the grains. Add soy sauce and bay leaf and bring to boil, then add the grains and cumin. Turn heat down to slow-boil until liquid is absorbed and grains are light and fluffy, 15 to 20 minutes. Transfer to a serving bowl by fluffing with a fork. Toss in pine nuts and parsley as you go, reserving a tablespoon of each for garnish.

To prepare sauce, place broth and soy sauce in a 1-quart saucepan and bring to boil. Turn heat down to medium. In a small bowl, dissolve thickener (kuzu or arrowroot) in cool water to barely cover and add to pot. Stir until mixture simmers, thickens, and becomes shiny, about 30 seconds. Allow to cool somewhat before serving to thicken further.

To serve, pour ¼-cup sauce to fill half of the plate. Pack a ½-cup stainless measuring cup once or twice with pilaf and tap to unmold the mound(s) on top of sauce. Garnish pilaf with a carrot cutout and a fresh green leaf.

SEASON'S GREENS AND RED RADISHES WITH CITRUS-FLAX OIL VINAIGRETTE

Makes 3 to 4 servings

> 1 bunch greens of the season, such as kale, collards, mustard, broccoli, broccoli rabe, sliced
> 1 bunch red radishes, halved or quartered
> water (1-2 inches for hardy greens such as kale, collard and mustard, depending on size of pot; ½ inch for broccoli)
> **Citrus-Flax Oil Vinaigrette: Makes ½ cup**
> ¼ cup combined lemon juice and brown rice vinegar
> 1-2 Tbsp combined extra virgin olive oil and flaxseed oil
> 1 Tbsp water
> ½ tsp sea salt
> freshly ground pepper
> 1 small clove garlic, pressed

Bring water to boil in a pot of appropriate size. Add greens, pressing to submerge hardy greens. Cook until tender, 5 to 7 minutes for kale and collards, 3 to 5 minutes for mustard and broccolis. Add radishes in last minute of cooking.

Meanwhile, mix dressing ingredients. Drain vegetables and dress lightly to serve.

ORGANIC FIELD GREEN SALAD WITH CANDIED ALMONDS AND SWEET MUSTARD-GARLIC VINAIGRETTE

> **Sweet Mustard-Garlic Vinaigrette: Makes ½ cup**
> 2 Tbsp brown rice vinegar
> 2 Tbsp brown rice syrup
> 1 Tbsp extra virgin olive oil
> 1 Tbsp water
> 1 Tbsp mustard
> 1 clove garlic, pressed
> ½ tsp sea salt
> **Candied Almonds or Almond Brittle: Makes ½ cup**
> ½ cup sliced almonds
> 2 Tbsp brown rice syrup
> **Salad**
> 8 cups mixed baby lettuces, about ½ lb, torn in large bite-size pieces

handful of sunflower sprouts (optional)

Whisk dressing ingredients together and allow to sit to meld flavors.

To prepare almonds, preheat oven to 300 degrees. In a dry pie pan, toast almonds until golden, about 8 minutes. In a bowl, mix almonds with sweetener. Line pan with parchment paper or brush it with oil and transfer almonds to pan. Bake until sweetener bubbles and is golden, about 15 minutes. Allow to cool in pan. Peel nuts from paper or scrape from pan with a spatula. Soak pan for ease in cleaning.

Toss the salad greens with the dressing just before serving. Garnish with nuts.

BRAISED TEMPEH WITH GREEN HERB COULIS
Makes 3 to 4 servings

You can make the coulis sauce a couple of days ahead. Color, flavor and consistency are maintained with refrigeration. A smaller volume is difficult to blend in a food processor.

> **Green Herb Coulis: Makes 3 to 5 servings or 1 to 1¼ cups**
>> **2 two-ounce bunches basil, 3 cups, leaves only**
>> **Up to 12 large sprigs mint, 2 ounces or 1½ cups, leaves only**
>> **2 large cloves garlic**
>> **2 Tbsp lemon juice**
>> **1 Tbsp extra virgin olive oil**
>> **½ tsp sea salt**
>> **½ tsp soy sauce**
>> **1 Tbsp water (optional)**
>
> **Braised Tempeh**
>> **2 tsp extra virgin olive oil**
>> **8 ounces tempeh, sliced in half to make 2 thick slabs, or in ½-inch diagonals**
>> **2 tsp natural soy sauce**
>> **⅓ to ½ cup water**
>> **small sprigs of mint for garnish**

To make coulis, process all ingredients except water until smooth, then and only if needed, add water gradually to texture desired.

To prepare tempeh, heat oil in a skillet over medium-low heat. Tempeh should fit snugly. Brown one side and then the other, about 5 minutes each side.

Mix soy sauce and water. Turn heat low to avoid spattering and pour liquid over tempeh. Cover until tempeh is cooked all the way through and liquid is completely absorbed, about 10 minutes more.

To serve, spread ¼ to ⅓ cup coulis on each plate and lay tempeh on top. Garnish with a small sprig of basil.

Meredith McCarty is a macrobiotic counselor and a vegan (dairy-free vegetarian) cooking instructor. As a holistic nutritionist (Diet Counselor and Nutrition Educator), she has consulted, taught and lectured internationally since 1977. Formerly the associate editor of Natural Health magazine, Meredith co-directed a macrobiotic center in northern California for 19 years, and has authored three cookbooks, American Macrobiotic Cuisine, Fresh from a Vegetarian Kitchen, *and* Sweet and Natural, *which won The Best Vegetarian Cookbook, World Cookbook Award. Meredith currently resides in the San Francisco Bay Area and may be contacted through her website,* www.healingcuisine. com.

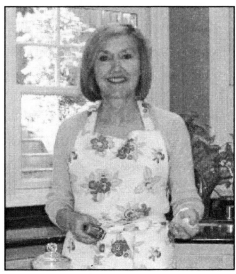

Meredith Teaching a Class

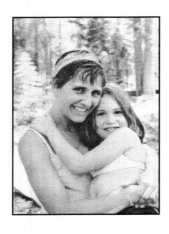

Recipes from

Dawn Pallavi

AREPAS

    1 cup water
    ¼ tsp unrefined sea salt, SI brand recommended
    1 to 2 tsp organic safflower oil
    2 cups organic masa flour
    1 medium organic onion, minced
    1 medium organic carrot, diced
    ¼ cup organic parsley, chopped
    2 organic scallions, cut into thin rounds
    organic safflower oil (to cover bottom of cast iron skillet)
    organic unpasteurized shoyu, to taste

Mix water, salt, and oil in a small bowl. Add this mixture to the masa flour and form into a dough. If the dough is too stiff, add 1 to 2 teaspoons more water. Mix the vegetables into the dough. Shape into croquettes. Heat oil in a cast iron skillet and pan fry the croquettes. When patties are browned on both sides, sprinkle a little shoyu on each patty and cook another minute on each side. Serve with Shoyu Ginger Dipping Sauce, Creamy Tofu Dip, or other sauce of choice.

    Variations: If you are starting with Homemade Corn Masa (in place of masa flour), you probably won't need to add any water to your previously prepared dough. Place patties on a parchment-lined baking sheet. Bake at 350 degrees F for 20 to 30 minutes or until golden brown. Sprinkle shoyu on each patty, to taste, during the last 10 minutes of cooking.

Add cilantro, Mexican oregano, cumin, or other herbs or spices of choice.

Tamale Filling

> 2 tsp organic sesame or olive oil
> 1 small organic yellow onion, diced
> 1 clove organic garlic, minced
> pinch unrefined sea salt, SI brand recommended
> ¼–½ tsp ground cumin, or to taste
> 1 small organic carrot, coarsely grated
> 1 cup organic seitan, tofu, or tempeh, finely diced (steam
>   tempeh 20 minutes before using)
> shoyu, to taste
> 2 Tbsp water

Lightly warm oil in a heavy skillet or Dutch oven. Sauté onion and garlic, adding sea salt and cumin to taste. Sauté until onion is transparent. Add carrot. Add seitan, tofu or tempeh and sauté 3–4 minutes, stirring well so that seasonings coat all of the ingredients. Season to taste with shoyu and if desired, add a few tablespoons of water to more evenly distribute the seasonings. Cook until no water is left, stirring continuously.

Tamales

In the Mexican culture, tamales are traditionally made by groups of families or friends for special occasions like Christmas and New Year's Eve.

> 6–12 corn husks
> warm water to cover
> 1 cup warm spring or filtered water (amount varies with brand of
>   masa)
> 1 tsp unrefined sea salt, SI brand recommended
> 5–6 Tbsp organic safflower oil (optional)
> 2 cups organic masa harina

Preparing Husks: Soak corn husks in warm water for about 1 hour. Drain in a basket just before forming tamales.

Dough: Mix water, salt, and oil in a bowl. Pour in masa harina, then mix with a spoon until a soft dough is formed. Knead lightly to mix evenly. Allow to rest while preparing other ingredients.

Filling: Prepare a filling of your choice and set aside. Puréed beans, sautéed vegetables, tofu, tempeh or seitan stir fries always work well. Season the filling well as the masa part of the tamale will be fairly bland. Ground cumin is a traditional seasoning used in Mexican and Southwestern cooking that works well in tamale fillings.

Forming Tamales: Lay 1 wide corn husk or 2 or 3 narrower ones on work surface. Dampen hands in a bowl of water. Take tennis ball sized piece of dough and form a ball. Press dough over corn husks to form a ¼-inch thick layer. The dough should go all the way to one side of the husk, but leave margins of ¼ inch at the top, 1½ inches at the bottom, and ½ inch on the other side.

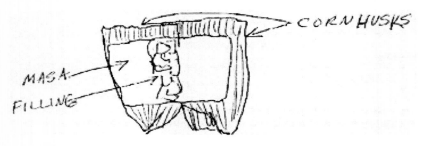

Put about 1 heaping tablespoon of filling down the center of the dough. Be careful not to overfill or the tamale will not close. Fold over so masa joins together with the filling in a column up the center of the tamale. Wrap the extra margin of corn husk around to seal the side and fold up the bottom ends to complete the casing.

Stand upright in a steamer and steam for 20–30 minutes until dough feels slightly bouncy and not too sticky. (You may need to steam for up to 60 minutes, depending on the filling and the number of tamales in the pot.)

Variations: Black beans—spiced with onions, garlic, Chinese 5 spice or cumin, red pepper, or hot mustard and maybe a minced jalapeño or serrano pepper—wrapped with masa is a terrific taste treat.

SALSA VERDE CRUDA (FRESH GREEN SALSA)
4 servings

> **2 cups water**
> **1 medium organic red onion, sliced ⅛ in thick**
> **¾ tsp organic black peppercorns, coarsely ground**
> **½ tsp organic dried oregano**
> **1 clove organic garlic, peeled and halved**
> **¼ cup organic ume vinegar**
> **¼ cup organic brown rice vinegar**
> **2 medium organic cucumbers**
> **1 organic avocado**
> **8 sprigs organic cilantro, chopped**
> **1 Tbsp organic ginger, peeled and finely chopped**
> **juice of 1 organic lime**
> **2 tsp organic umeboshi paste**

Pickled onions: Bring water to boil. Cook onion in boiling water for 1 minute. Remove onions to a jar or glass container for storage. Save 1 cup of cooking water, discard the rest, and set aside.

Coarsely grind peppercorns in a mortar then add to saucepan. Add the oregano, garlic, and vinegars to saucepan. Bring to a boil and turn heat off. Add ½ cup of poaching liquid to vinegar mixture. Pour hot liquid over onions in jar. Cover when completely cooled. These can be made ahead of time and stored in a covered jar until ready to use.

Salsa: Peel cucumbers and remove all of seeds, save seeds and put aside. Cut cucumbers into a small dice. Place cut cucumbers in a bowl.

Peel avocado and dice into small pieces and add to bowl.

Remove ½ pickled red onion from jar. Dice into small pieces and add to bowl. Do not rinse off spices. Add chopped cilantro, ginger, and juice of lime to bowl and mix well. Place half of your mixture in a food processor with ½ of cucumber seeds, ume paste, and ½ cup of poaching liquid. Process until smooth.

Add puréed half of salsa to mixture and mix well. Taste for salt and adjust with ume vinegar. Allow flavors to marinate for an hour before serving.

Variations: Pickle a chile with onions to add spicier flavor to salsa. Or, add mango, pineapple, or jicama to salsa for exotic flavors.

Dawn Pallavi is an experienced instructor and chef of natural foods who specializes in incorporating health and wellness into the culinary arts. She serves as Director and teaches cooking and nutrition at the Natural Epicurean Academy of Culinary Arts. With culinary training in France and the United States, Dawn brings a uniquely comprehensive perspective to the art of cooking and nutrition. She studies and teaches not only how to make natural foods look and taste great, but how those foods affect our lives, our moods, and our bodies. Through lectures, seminars, and cooking classes, she helps people reclaim their peak health and realize their dreams. Dawn has attended camp a number of times with her daughter, Joy. Visit her website at: www.naturalepicurean. com.

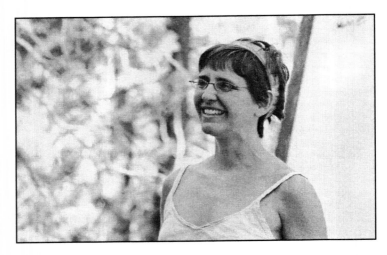

Dawn teaching at the 2006 French Meadows Camp

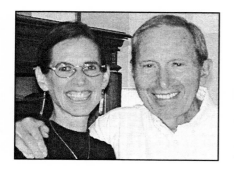

Recipes from

Ginat and Sheldon Rice

MORNING CEREAL

A delicious morning porridge can be made by pressure cooking or boiling rice, millet, barley, or other grain. Use 3 to 5 cups of water to 1 cup of grain. You may season it with salt or shoyu, or give it a sweet taste with dried fruit, apple juice, or grain sweetener. One cup of grain serves about 4 people.

Tips: Soaking energizes rice. Soak rice overnight to make porridge; soak 2 to 4 hours for lunch or supper. Do not add fire slowly to unsoaked rice; it makes it too yang. Rather, bring it to a boil over high heat.

Salt makes rice sweet and easier to digest. Use more salt in a damp climate than dry. Add salt after the rice comes to a boil.

Old rice may be energized by sautéing it with a small amount of sesame oil. Add shoyu to balance the oil.

Pressure cooking grains keeps in more nutrients, creates more energy in the food, is tastier, and makes the food easier to digest. Pressure cook for 50 minutes in the winter; 45 minutes in hot weather.

Rice and millet are the only grains without a split kernel. They help promote holistic thinking.

RICE CREAM

This soothing rice cream can be made in advance for several servings. We enjoy it on cold winter mornings, or when we're a bit under the weather. It is especially recommended in the following situations: Breaking a fast; digestion or chewing difficulties; low appetite or vitality; illness, including in children; and weakness.

½ cup organic brown rice
5 cups of water
Pinch of sea salt

Dry-roast ½ cup of organic brown rice over a medium heat until golden brown. Add 5 cups of water and bring to a boil; then add a pinch of salt. Cover and cook for about two hours over a heat diffuser on a low heat until the water is about ½ the original amount.

Alternately, cook in a pressure cooker for 1 hour with 2½ cups of water. Let the rice cool and then squeeze it out through cotton cheesecloth. Reheat the liquid as needed to serve.

Mixed Media Summer Salad

This salad combines several different cooking styles, giving it energy and flair. It is simple yet varied—a winning combination.

spaghetti, cooked a bit more than al dente; rinsed
broccoli and red onion, blanched
fresh lettuce and arugula
radish slices long-cooked in ume paste
cauliflower, steamed
crushed roasted sesame seed paste with water

Mix all these ingredients together in a big bowl. Top with boiled, mashed tofu mixed with chopped sauerkraut.

Variations: Vegetable Noodle Adzuki Bean Salad—add beans to the basic recipe. Buckwheat Salad—substitute this or any grain for the spaghetti. Steamed broccoli or any other vegetable instead of the cauliflower.

Grated Carrot Salad with Sweet Rice Vinegar
Serves 4

This simple and delicious salad is a pleasure to serve when you see the delight on your guests' faces. It's a taste treat that is ready in moments. Use a round porcelain grater for easiest grating.

2 cups carrots, finely grated
3 Tbsp sweet brown rice vinegar

Toss the finely grated carrots with the vinegar. Allow the mixture to marinate about 30 minutes before serving. Toss occasionally while marinating to ensure that the flavors blend evenly. Serve at room temperature.

WAKAME-CUCUMBER SALAD

This delicious salad is a macrobiotic standard and a hit every time. Its light, upward energy is refreshing all year round, and the addition of tangerine slices gives it a special appeal.

> **1 cup water**
> **1 cup sliced soaked wakame**
> **2 cups cucumbers, halved and sliced**
> **1 tangerine**
> **1 Tbsp soy sauce**
> **1 Tbsp sweet brown rice vinegar**
> **fresh ginger**

Add wakame to a small amount of boiling water and simmer for 1 to 2 minutes. If it still seems hard, cook 3 to 5 minutes. Drain the wakame and allow to cool. Alternately, use instant (*Isa*) wakame, and no cooking is necessary—just soak the flakes for a few minutes and strain out the liquid.

Slice the cucumbers thinly and mix with the wakame in a bowl. Cut the tangerine into cubes, de-seed, and mix with the cucumbers and wakame. Press for ½ to 1 hour, and then drain off the expressed liquid.

Make a sauce by mixing together shoyu, vinegar, and a small amount of grated ginger juice. Mix with the salad.

Sheldon and Ginat Rice are long-time macrobiotic teachers and counselors. They have attended several French Meadows Camps and always enjoy the chance to try out new recipes on open-wood fires. They spearhead the macrobiotic community in Israel where they operate a macrobiotic Bed & Breakfast from their home in Jerusalem. Visit www. TheRiceHouse.com; *call 9722-566-9367; or e-mail* shelgin@netvision. net.il.

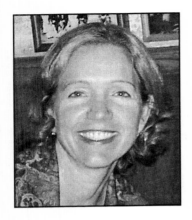

Recipes from

Laura Stec

FRESH HERB COUSCOUS

> 1 cup mixed chopped herbs, such as parsley, basil, chives and
>   tarragon
> 1 large garlic clove, quartered
> 2-3 tsp olive oil
> 1¼ cups boiling water
> 1 cup couscous (white or wheat)
> ½ tsp salt

In a mini food processor or blender, combine the herbs, garlic, olive oil, and ¼ cup of the boiling water and process to a paste.

Place couscous in a 8 inch square pan. Mix remaining water with herb mixture and pour over couscous. Cover and let sit for 10 minutes until water is absorbed. Fluff with fork and serve.

OVEN-ROASTED WINTER ROOT VEGETABLES

> 1 lb root vegetables of your choice: potatoes, rutabagas,
>   turnips, sweet potatoes
> a few cloves garlic, peeled
> olive oil
> salt
> 1 Tbsp fresh rosemary – chopped (optional)

Preheat oven to 375 degrees F. Cut vegetables into ¾-inch chunks. Rub with olive oil and sprinkle with salt. Add chopped rosemary. Bake until tender, approximately 1 hour. Serve.

TEMPEH, MUSHROOM, AND CELERY FRICASSEE
6 servings

> 1 Tbsp olive oil
> 12 oz tempeh, cut into ½ inch cubes
> ¼ cup veggie stock or white wine
> 2 Tbsp soy sauce
> ½ cup celery, sliced
> 4 cups thinly sliced leek (about 4 large)
> 2 cups sliced shiitake mushrooms
> 2 cups sliced button mushrooms
> 2 cups sliced cremini mushrooms
> 1 Tbsp whole wheat pastry flour
> 2 thyme sprigs
> 1 parsley sprig
> 5 garlic cloves, thinly sliced
> 1 (14.5 oz) can veggie stock
> 1 Tbsp lemon juice
> ¼ tsp salt
> ¼ tsp black pepper
> 2 Tbsp chopped parsley
> 1 Tbsp grated lemon rind

Heat a sauté pan, add oil and tempeh; sauté 8 minutes or until golden brown. Add stock or wine and soy sauce, cook 15 seconds or until liquid almost evaporates. Remove tempeh from pan. Add celery to pan, sauté 5 minutes. Add leeks and mushrooms, sauté 5 minutes. Stir in flour, cook 1 minute. Add herbs, garlic and broth to pan, bring to a boil. Add tempeh, stirring well. Cover, reduce heat and simmer 15 minutes.

Uncover and cook 3 minutes or until thick. Discard herbs. Stir in lemon juice, salt and pepper; sprinkle with parsley. Garnish each serving with ½ teaspoon lemon rind, if desired.

GRILLED VEGETABLES

Using vegetables of your choice, slice into "grillable" sizes and marinate in Basic Marinade for ½ hour. Grill until tender.

Note: to save grilling time you may want to quick blanch harder veggies like carrots and cauliflower.

BASIC MARINADE

Use for roasted or grilled veggies.

Measure equal parts balsamic vinegar, olive oil, soy sauce. For variety, add favorite herbs and spices: Asian dishes add toasted sesame oil and lemongrass. Southwestern dishes add cumin and cilantro. Italian dishes add fresh oregano and basil.

FLAX SUNFLOWER BASIL UMEBOSHI GOMASIO

1 cup sunflower seed
4 tsp umeboshi vinegar
1 cup flax seeds, ground
2 tsp dried basil
2-2½ Tbsp salt

Preheat oven to 350 degrees F. Roast sunflower seeds on a baking sheet for 7 minutes. Toss with umeboshi vinegar and return to oven for 2 minutes. Remove from oven. Put sunflower seeds, flax, basil, and salt in food processor and grind until smooth. Sprinkle on whole grains.

THREE GRAIN PILAF
6 servings

1 Tbsp olive oil
½ cup green onions, chopped
1 cup uncooked brown basmati rice
½ cup uncooked quinoa
½ cup uncooked millet
3 cups veggie broth
¼ tsp salt

Heat sauce pot, add oil and green onions, cook 1 minute. Wash grains and add to pot, cook 3 minutes, stirring frequently. Stir in broth and salt. Bring to a boil, reduce heat, cover and cook for 40 minutes.

Laura Stec headed the French Meadows kitchen in 1998 and 1999 and was instrumental in the transition of the kitchen from Cornellia Aihara to the next generation. Laura is a whole foods chef, instructor, environmental leader and author, trained at the Culinary Institute of America, Vega Study Center, and the School of Natural Cookery. Laura Stec — Innovative Cuisine is her personal chef and education business. She is Culinary Health Instructor at Kaiser Permanente Medical Centers for Healthwords (corporate wellness), weight loss and Lifestyle programs, as well as the former chef for Kaiser's organic farmer's market. She is former chef instructor for LifeLong Inc. (a medical weight-loss program) and teaches all over the San Francisco Bay area. Laura is also a long-time staff member with environmental organization, Acterra and is passionate about educating on the connections between food choices and the environment. She is author of The Global Warming Diet - Cool Recipes for a Hot Planet *with atmospheric scientist Dr. Eugene Cordero of San Jose State University. Their book will be released in 2008. See:* www.globalwarmingdiet.org *or* www.laurastec.com.

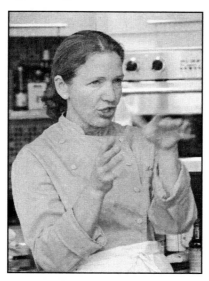

Laura Teaching a Class

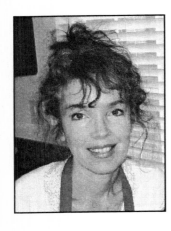

Recipes from
Lisa Valantine

STRAWBERRY COUSCOUS CAKE

Cake:
> 2 cups whole wheat couscous
> 3 cups almond amasake
> 1 cup water
> ½ cup apple juice
> pinch sea salt
> 2 tsp vanilla extract

Topping:
> 2 heaping Tbsp kuzu
> 1½ cups apple juice
> 1 tsp grated organic lemon peel
> ½ tsp vanilla extract
> 2½ cups fresh sliced strawberries

Cake: Combine couscous, amasake, water, juice, and sea salt in a saucepan. Bring up to heat and cook for 10 minutes, stirring often until couscous is soft and cooked. Remove from heat. Stir in vanilla extract. Pour mixture into a 9 x 13 Pyrex baking pan. Smooth the surface of the cake with a rubber spatula.

Topping: Dissolve kuzu in the juice and heat until the mixture thickens. Add lemon peel and vanilla. Pour the topping over the cake. Arrange the strawberries. Let cool for about an hour before serving.

APPLESAUCE PUDDING

3 cups organic applesauce
3 cups organic apple juice
pinch sea salt
3 Tbsp kuzu
½ tsp grated organic lemon rind
1 tsp vanilla
handful toasted almond slivers
handful currants

Bring the applesauce, 2 cups apple juice, and sea salt to a boil. While applesauce is coming to a boil, dissolve kuzu in the remaining 1 cup of apple juice. Once the applesauce is boiling carefully stir in the dissolved kuzu. Cook until the kuzu turns clear. Add lemon rind and vanilla. Serve in individual cups with a garnish of almonds and currants. Serve at room temperature.

Lisa Valantine lives in the Los Angles area where she offers nutritional consulting, classes, and cooking. She has attended a number of camps and one year, presented a cooking class on desserts. We are pleased to share these recipes. To contact Lisa, call 805-371-8907.

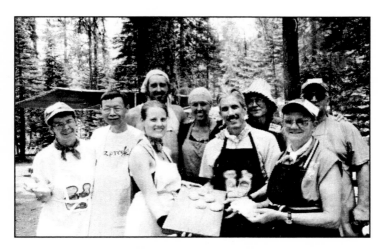

Chuck's Bread Baking Experience Class at the 2002
French Meadows Camp

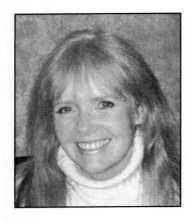

Recipes from
Melanie Waxman

EUROPEAN FRIED RICE

>1 Tbsp olive oil (optional)
>1 onion, diced
>2 cloves garlic, sliced (optional)
>½ cup round cabbage, rinsed and shredded
>1 carrot, washed and grated
>1 cup cooked chickpeas, can use a can of organic chickpeas
>2 cups brown rice, cooked
>½ cups spring water
>1 tsp sea salt

Warm skillet over high heat for a few seconds and add oil. Use water instead of oil if desired. Add the onion and garlic (optional) to the oil and sauté for a few minutes. Add the cabbage and sauté a further minute. Add the carrot and continue to sauté for another minute. Add the chickpeas and mix through the vegetables.

Place the cooked rice on top of the vegetables. Add the water and season with salt. Cook on low heat, with a lid, for about 5 minutes. Mix the rice and vegetables together and serve from the skillet.

CARROT DAIKON CONDIMENT

>1 Tbsp finely grated carrot
>1 Tbsp finely grated daikon
>½ tsp shiso powder

few drops shoyu
fresh lemon juice

Place the ingredients in a bowl and mix gently. Serve on top of rice.

WATERCRESS SALAD

Serves: 2-4 people
Preparation time: 10 minutes

2 cups daikon, finely sliced into matchsticks
sea salt
½ cup spring water
2 fresh shiitake, finely sliced
1 tsp shoyu
½ tsp orange rind
1 tsp mirin
1 bunch watercress, sliced
½ cup sesame seeds, toasted
1 tsp umeboshi vinegar
½ Granny Smith apple, finely sliced

Place the daikon on a plate. Mix with a little sea salt. Place another plate and weight on top of the daikon. Leave for about 15 minutes.

Place the water, shiitake, shoyu, orange rind, and mirin in a pan. Cover with a lid. Bring to a boil and simmer about 10 minutes. Add the watercress and cook a further 30 seconds. Remove and place on a serving plate.

Grind the sesame seeds to a fine powder and add the umeboshi vinegar. Place the shiitake, blanched watercress, and sliced apple in a serving dish. Add the pressed daikon and sesame seeds. Toss gently and serve.

STUFFED CUCUMBERS

¼ block firm tofu, mashed
1 tsp umeboshi vinegar
1 tsp finely diced roasted red pepper, can be purchased in a jar
1 tsp capers
1 European cucumber, peeled
1 tsp chives, finely chopped

Mix the tofu, umeboshi vinegar, pepper, and capers. Scoop out the seeds from the cucumber. Stuff the cucumber with the tofu mixture. Let sit for about 20 minutes. Slice into bite-size pieces and serve garnished with chopped chives.

Well-known macrobiotic teacher, Melanie Waxman has worked with clients and students from all over the world, including the famous Boy George. Her studies in Oriental medicine began in the 1980s and she went on to specialize in Feng Shui, macrobiotic cooking, coaching, writing, and massage. Melanie has lived in England, Portugal, and the United States. Her written works include a series of 12 Upbeat Macrobiotic Cooklets that are used worldwide, Mr. Hoppity's Color Me Cookbook for Kids, Bless the Baby *(published by Carroll and Brown) and* Yummy Yummy in My Tummy. *She also writes for numerous magazines and web sites and has been quoted in* British Vogue *and* Woman's Own. *Melanie currently maintains an active alternative health practice in Chester County, Pennsylvania. Her new book* Eat Me Now! *is now available.*

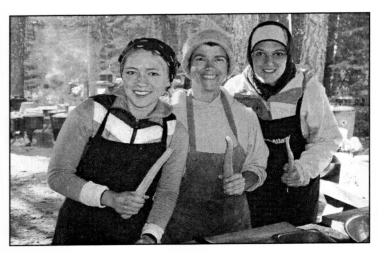

Heather, Missy, and Beth Preparing Carrots at the 2007 French Meadows Camp

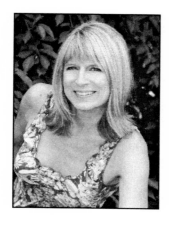

Recipes from

Susan Waxman

BOILED DAIKON WITH SWEET MISO SAUCE

daikon cut on the diagonal, into ½- to ¾-inch slices
sea salt
water
sweet tasting brown rice miso
roasted tahini
brown rice syrup

Place cut daikon in a pot with water to cover and a small pinch of sea salt. Cover and bring to a boil on a medium-high heat. Lower the heat and simmer until the daikon is tender—approximately 30 to 40 minutes depending the thickness and texture of the daikon.

While the daikon is cooking prepare the sauce. Place 1 slightly rounded teaspoon of miso in a bowl and dilute with a few drops of the daikon cooking water; mix well. Add 2 teaspoons of tahini and blend together with the miso. Add 2 teaspoons of brown rice syrup; stir well until all ingredients are blended into a thick sauce.

When the daikon is thoroughly cooked place each piece on a flat serving platter and allow to cool for a minute before adding the sauce. Place a small amount of sauce on each piece of daikon and serve immediately, while hot.

Option: Garnish with toasted black sesame seeds.

FRIED COUSCOUS—RED ONION, CARROT, PEAS

2 cups water
sea salt
1 cup of couscous
light sesame oil or olive oil
½ cup of onion, diced
1/3 cup of carrot, diced
1/3 cup of green peas
shoyu
1/3 cup of finely chopped parsley
ume vinegar

Place the water and sea salt in a pot and bring to a boil. Add couscous to the boiling water. Cover, lower heat, and let sit for 5 minutes. Remove from the pot and place in a bowl.

Heat a skillet and add the oil. Add the onion and sauté. Add a pinch of salt. Add the carrots and green peas and continue to sauté. Season the vegetables with a few drops of shoyu. Mix vegetables with the couscous. Add chopped parsley and several drops of ume vinegar and mix well. Place in a serving bowl and cover.

Option: Substitute cooked chickpeas for the green peas. For a heartier dish add finely chopped seitan.

CORN FRITTERS

This recipe was adapted from my mother's Pennsylvania Dutch recipe.

1-2 ears of corn
1 cup unbleached flour
¼ teaspoon sea salt
2 Tbsp of olive oil
1 tsp umeboshi paste
2 Tbsp brown rice syrup
fizzy water
oil for pan frying

Use a round porcelain grater to finely 1 to 2 ears of corn—enough to make ½ cup. Place dry ingredients in a bowl and mix with a fork.

In a separate bowl blend the olive oil, ume paste, and rice syrup together. Make a well in the middle of the dry ingredients and add the wet ingredients. Add the corn and blend all ingredients together. Add fizzy water gradually, up to ¼ cup, to make a thick batter. A helpful hint: the batter should be a "sticky" consistency.

Pan fry in a cast iron skillet. Use oil appropriate for high temperature frying. Add enough oil to cover the bottom of the pan by ½ an inch. Allow the oil to heat before you begin frying. Use a spoon to place the batter in the pan. Fry until the fritter turns a golden brown. Place on a paper towel to drain off any excess oil.

Susan Waxman has been a macrobiotic teacher and counselor for sixteen years. As co-director of The Strengthening Health Institute (SHI) in Philadelphia, PA, a center dedicated to macrobiotic education, whose goal is the promotion of personal and planetary health, Susan has devoted herself to the advancement of the macrobiotic way of dietary health, exercise, and life style. Susan has a BA in Psychology, Sociology and Anthropology from the University of Pittsburgh. Before dedicating her life to macrobiotics, she worked in the field of Social Services, primarily with children and young adults.

Susan's personal passion is the art of cooking. As executive chef of the Genmai Café she is widely recognized for her culinary expertise, as well as her understanding of the energetic properties of food. Susan's innovative style and attention to detail shows through in the flavor and healing power of her food. In addition to sessions offered in Philadelphia, Susan also travels with her husband, Denny Waxman, offering seminars throughout the U.S. and Europe. Susan can be contacted at www.strengthenhealth.org.

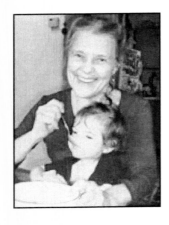

Recipes from

Rebecca Wood

THREE SISTER SOUP

My favorite soup is composed of the new world's staple trinity—posole, beans, and squash.

> ¾ cup dry posole
> ½ cup anasazi or pinto beans
> 2 Tbsp sesame oil or ghee
> 1 tsp cumin seed
> 2 cloves minced garlic
> 1 chopped, large onion
> 1½ cups chopped butternut or kabocha squash
> 1 New Mexican chile, blistered, steamed, peeled, seeded, and diced
> ⅓ cup (loosely packed) sea palm
> 1 bay leaf
> 2 tsp sea salt
> 5 cups water
> lime juice to taste
> ¼ cup chopped fresh epazote or cilantro

Soak the posole and beans in water to cover overnight. In a large soup pot, warm the oil and lightly sauté the cumin, garlic, onion, squash, and chile. Drain the posole. Add posole, beans, sea palm, bay leaf, and water to the pot, cover, bring to a boil, reduce heat, and simmer for one hour. Add salt and continue cooking until the posole "butterflies" open and the beans are tender. Season to taste with fresh lime juice. Garnish generously with cilantro or epazote.

THE ONLY MAIN COURSE SALAD RECIPE YOU NEED

Here's a basic formula for an endless variety of one-dish meals that also pack well for lunches. For a side dish, reduce the quantity of grains or beans. If you use already seasoned grains or beans, dress the salad with the same flavors. If you use black beans, rinse them until the water runs clear or their liquid will discolor the other ingredients. This substantial salad welcomes a more liberal amount of either vinegar, lemon juice or ume vinegar than does a lighter green salad. Tasty optional ingredients include: cooked sweet corn, cooked and cubed chicken breast, snow peas, fresh herbs, olives or sun-dried tomatoes.

> **2 cups cooked grain, pasta or beans of choice**
> **1 diced carrot**
> **2 stalks chopped celery or fennel**
> **½ diced red or green bell pepper**
> **2 to 4 sliced scallions or finely chopped red onion**
> **¼ cup toasted nuts or sunflower seeds**
> **¼ cup salad dressing of choice**

Combine salad ingredients, dress and allow to rest for 10 minutes. Taste and adjust seasoning. Serve on a bed of lettuce. Serves 2 as a main course.

STEAMED AMARANTH

The robust, peppery flavor and chewy texture of tiny amaranth seeds are unlike any other grain. This high protein grain imparts more energy than the common grains.

> **1 cup amaranth**
> **1½ cups water**
> **⅛ tsp sea salt**

Toast amaranth in a saucepan, stirring continuously, for 3 to 4 minutes or until the amaranth turns a shade darker and a few of the grains pop. Add water and salt. Cover, bring to a boil, reduce heat and simmer for about 15 minutes or until the liquid is absorbed. Makes about 2 cups.

WAYFARER'S BREAD

When cooked and cooled, amaranth's minuscule grains stick together enabling you to flatten and cook it into a tortilla-like bread which is crisp on the outside, but soft and moist inside. It's an unusual—but satisfying—texture. The thinner you press the bread, the crisper the result. Serve this flat bread with vegetable soup for a light meal or pack it for lunch.

> 1 Tbsp unrefined sesame oil or ghee
> 1 tsp sesame seeds
> 2 cups cooked and cooled amaranth

Warm the oil in an 8-inch crepe or sauté pan over medium heat. Add sesame seeds and sauté for 30 seconds or until aromatic.

Scrape the amaranth into the pan and press the amaranth into a ⅛-inch thickness to form a 6-inch diameter bread. Cook for 5 minutes or until the edges start to dry and slightly curl up and the bottom is browned. Turn and cook the other side for 4 minutes or until browned. Remove to a cutting board. When cooled enough to work with, slice into pie-shaped wedges and serve warm or cold.

SARRASIN CREPES
Makes 12, 7-inch crepes

Here's a light but satisfying breakfast crepe that is delicious with syrup or jam for breakfast, or for lunch entrée, roll a savory filing into it.

> 1 cup buckwheat flour
> 2 Tbsp wheat or barley flour
> 1 tsp ground coriander
> ⅛ tsp sea salt
> 1¾ cups water
> 2 large eggs
> ¼ cup melted unsalted butter, cooled

Combine dry ingredients. Whisk together water, eggs and 2 tablespoons butter. When blended, stir half of this into the flour, mixing until no longer lumpy. Stir in the remaining liquid to form a smooth batter. Set aside for 15 minutes.

Heat a 7-inch crepe pan, brush it with some of the remaining butter, and grasp the pan in one hand. Fill a ¼ cup measure with batter and pour the batter onto the pan while rotating the pan so that a thin layer of batter covers its surface. Return the pan to the heat. Cook for 2 to 3 minutes or until the top dries. Turn and cook an additional minute or until the bottom is lightly browned. Repeat until all the batter is used, keeping the cooked crepes warm. Serve warm topped with a fruit sauce, jam, or honey.

TWELVE-LAYER FRENCH MEADOWS CAKE

This festive dessert is a great celebratory activity for a small group. Heat up every available skillet, one person flips crepes, another slices fruit, someone chops nuts, another whips cream, and then many hands contribute to the layering of cake, cream, fruit and the spontaneous decorating.

> **12 buckwheat crepes (Sarrasin Crepes)**
> **6 cups firm seasonal fruit such as berries, apples, pears, or peaches**
> **3 cups whipped cream (or thick vanilla pudding)**
> **1 cup roasted, chopped walnuts**

Unless the fruit is small—like berries—cut into small pieces (large chunks of fruit make a cake that's hard to stack). Place one crepe on a serving platter, add a layer of fruit, a second crepe, a layer of cream and continue building until all the ingredients are used. Slice into wedges and serve immediately.

Rebecca Wood is an award-winning author of The Splendid Grain *that won both a James Beard Award and a Julia Child/IACP Cookbook Award. Rebecca attended camp a number of times, from the early days in 1970 to more recently in 1998 and 1999. Currently she lives in Ward, Colorado where she counsels and is revising* The New Whole Foods Encyclopedia *to be published by Penguin in 2009. Her website,* www. rwood.com, *contains many recipes, articles, and a forum.*

Cornellia's Menus

Cornellia Aihara established the kitchen tradition at French Meadows in 1970 and faithfully cooked for many years. In 1979, she published her cookbook, Calendar Cookbook, which contains a log of menus from 1972, including the menus she served at French Meadows camp. On the next page is a reprint of those brunches and dinners.

At my (J.F.) first summer camp in 1981, Cornellia served a similar menu. Every day brunch was at 11:30 and dinner at 5:30. Many of the selections were the same, notably azuki bean rice and fresh corn on the first evening's menu, and tempura dinner on the last. One thing had changed, and that was the inclusion of breakfast at 7:30 am. By 1981, Cornellia served oatmeal to children, nursing mothers, pregnant women, and anyone unable to fast until brunch. By her last camp, 1997, this had changed too, as Cornellia was serving breakfast to everyone.

One feature that identifies Cornellia's tradition at camp is that she served a standard type menu every day—in particular, pressure-cooked brown rice, miso soup, cooked vegetables, nuka pickles, and tea for brunch; pressure-cooked brown rice, a soup other than miso soup, nuka pickles, and an assortment of other dishes such as bean dishes, sea vegetable dishes, and desserts for dinner. Many of her recipes are presently served at camp; most of her tradition remains, as the current menu always includes a grain dish, vegetables, soup, and pickles.

Friday, August 17, 1972

Breakfast
Wakame, onion, cabbage miso soup
Pressure-cooked brown rice
Baked rice balls with tamari
Cucumber nuka pickles

Dinner
Azuki bean rice
Summer vegetable macaroni soup
Corn on the cob, outdoor cooking
Crookneck squash, onion nitsuke
Chinese cabbage nuka pickles

Saturday, August 18, 1972

Breakfast
Vegetable miso soup with buckwheat
    dumplings
Pressure-cooked brown rice
Mustard green, onion nitsuke
Hijiki, carrot nitsuke
Cucumber, daikon leaves nuka pickles

Dinner
Pressure-cooked brown rice
Vegetables with kuzu sauce
Nori nitsuke
Tossed salad with French dressing

Sunday, August 19, 1972

Breakfast
Turnip, onion, carrot miso soup
Pressure-cooked brown rice
Saifun nitsuke
Top of stove bread with pear butter
Cucumber nuka pickles

Dinner
Pressure-cooked brown rice
Lentil soup
Pan-fried whole wheat spaghetti
Boiled beets
Chinese cabbage nuka pickles

Monday, August 20, 1972

Breakfast
Wakame, onion, cabbage miso soup
Pressure-cooked brown rice
Rice cream
Summer squash nitsuke
Watermelon

Dinner
Pressure-cooked brown rice
Split pea macaroni soup
Onion miso
Cucumber, cabbage nuka pickles

Tuesday, August 21, 1972

Breakfast
Barley miso soup
Pressure-cooked brown rice
Tekka miso
String bean, celery nitsuke with
    sesame butter
Watermelon rind nuka pickles

Dinner
Pressure-cooked brown rice
Polenta potage with whole wheat
    noodle salad with sesame
    butter dressing
Dried daikon nitsuke
Cabbage, celery nuka pickles

Wednesday, August 22, 1972

Breakfast
Cabbage, onion, carrot miso soup
Pressure-cooked brown rice
Butternut squash, onion nitsuke
    with polenta potage (leftover)
Dried daikon nitsuke (leftover)
Celery, cabbage nuka pickles
Watermelon

Dinner
Gomoku rice
Egg drop soup
Saifun salad with mayonnaise
    dressing

Thursday, August 23, 1972

Breakfast
Onion, turnip, carrot miso soup
Pressure-cooked brown rice
Sweet potato, carrot nitsuke
Nori, kombu nitsuke
Chinese cabbage nuka pickles

Dinner
Pressure-cooked brown rice
Vegetables with curry sauce
Scallion miso
Chinese cabbage nuka pickles

Friday, August 24, 1972

Breakfast
Onion, cabbage, crookneck squash
    miso soup
Pressure-cooked brown rice
Broiled beets with tops
String bean nitsuke with sesame
    butter
Cucumber nuka pickles
Watermelon

Dinner
Pressure-cooked brown rice
Buckwheat noodles with clear
    soup
Hijiki, onion nitsuke
Tossed salad

Saturday, August 25, 1972

Breakfast

Buckwheat dumpling miso soup
Pressure-cooked brown rice
Zucchini onion nitsuke
Watermelon rind nuka pickles

Dinner

Azuki bean rice
Clear soup with cucumber
Vegetable tempura
Grated daikon and carrot
Ohitashi
Apple–pear kanten

Sunday, August 26, 1972

Breakfast

Butternut squash, onion miso soup
Pressure-cooked brown rice
Vegetable tempura (leftover)
Creamed cabbage
Watermelon rind nuka pickles

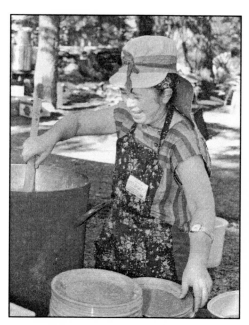

**Cornellia Serving at the 1997
French Meadows Camp**

Current Menus

FIRST THURSDAY — "CAMP SET-UP DAY"

BREAKFAST
Main Grain	Oatmeal
Second Grain	Toast
Seeds/Nuts	Sunflower seeds
	Peanut butter
Sweet Source	Raisins
Salt Source	Gomashio

LUNCH
Main Grain	Brown rice
Second Grain	Soba with scallion and nori garnish
Protein Source	Fried tempeh
Fat Source	Roasted walnuts with soy sauce, garnish
Soup/Bowl	Kombu and shiitake clear broth with soy sauce
Vegetable Dish	Broccoli with walnut sprinkle
	Kombu, shiitake, soy sauce condiment
Sea Vegetables	(nori in garnish and kombu in clear broth)
Pickle or Sour	Gomashio

SNACK   Cantaloupe

DINNER
Main Grain	Brown rice
Protein Source	(lentils in soup)
Fat Source	(tahini in dressing)
Soup/Bowl	Lentil soup
Vegetable Dish	Corn on the cob
	Blanched radish greens
	Salad-leaf lettuce with radishes, celery, carrot
	Dressing: umeboshi, lemon juice, tahini
Pickle or Sour	Dill pickle
	(ume and lemon in dressing)

FIRST FRIDAY — "FIRST DAY OF CAMP" "TRANSITION DAY"

BREAKFAST
Main Grain	Oatmeal
Second Grain	Toast
Seeds/Nuts	Peanut butter
Sweet Source	Apple butter
Salt Source	Gomashio

LUNCH
Main Grain	Brown rice
Second Grain	Pasta with blanched kale, onion, Chinese cabbage, yellow squash, carrot and chickpeas
Protein Source	(chickpeas)
Fat Source	Tahini sauce
Soup/Bowl	Barley miso soup with wakame, winter squash, bok choy, scallion
Vegetable Dish	(vegetables in soup and noodle dish)
Sea Vegetables	(wakame in soup)
Pickle or Sour	Dill pickle
Extra Dish	Gomashio

SNACK   Cantaloupe

DINNER   Cornellia Aihara's Menu
Main Grain	Brown rice with azuki beans
Second Grain	(oatmeal in soup)
Protein Source	(azuki in rice)
Fat Source	(olive oil in dressing and sesame oil in soup/arame)
Soup/Bowl	Creamy onion soup with onions, oatmeal, celery, rice miso
Vegetable Dish	Corn on the cob
	Salad—leaf lettuce with red cabbage, jicama, and blanched snow peas
	Dressing: ume, red onion, olive oil, lemon, dill
Sea Vegetables	Arame with carrots and sauteed onion
Pickle or Sour	Dill pickle (ume and lemon in dressing)
Fruit/Dessert	Peach kanten
Salty Condiment	Gomashio

FIRST SATURDAY — "FIRST FULL DAY FOR MANY CAMPERS" "SET RHYTHM"

BREAKFAST
Main Grain	Oatmeal
Second Grain	Toast
Seeds/Nuts	Pumpkin seeds
Sweet Source	Apple butter
Salt Source	Gomashio

LUNCH
Main Grain	Brown rice salad with almonds
Second Grain	(noodle in soup)
Protein Source	(almonds)
Fat Source	(dressing for salad and almonds in sprinkle)
	(almonds)
Soup/Bowl	Barley miso soup with sauteed onion, wakame, cabbage, scallion, noodles
Vegetable Dish	Kale
Sea Vegetables	(wakame in soup)
Pickle or Sour	Dill pickle
Salty Condiment	Gomashio

SNACK   Watermelon

DINNER
Main Grain	Brown rice
Second Grain	Corn chips with salsa
Protein Source	(black beans)
Fat Source	(salad dressing)
Soup/Bowl	Black bean soup
Vegetable Dish	Corn on the cob
	Salad—romaine lettuce, carrot, cucumber, and red cabbage
	Dressing: olive oil and ume vinegar
Pickle or Sour	Dill pickle
Salty Condiment	Gomashio

FIRST SUNDAY — "IN THE GROOVE DAY"

BREAKFAST
Main Grain	Millet with amaranth
Second Grain	Oatmeal
Seeds/Nuts	Sunflower seeds
Sweet Source	Apple/raisin/pear relish
Salt Source	Gomashio

LUNCH
Main Grain	Brown rice pups rolled in gomashio
Second Grain	Curry noodle salad with corn, carrot, and cucumbers
Protein Source	
Fat Source	(dressings)
Soup/Bowl	Barley miso soup with wakame and bok choy
Vegetable Dish	Chinese cabbage roll
Sea Vegetables	Wakame cucumber salad
Pickle or Sour	Dill pickle
Extra Dish	Gomashio

SNACK   Watermelon

DINNER
Main Grain	Brown rice, long grain
Second Grain	Polenta
Protein Source	Pinto beans
Fat Source	Black olives, (tahini in dressing)
Soup/Bowl	(only if pinto beans are soupy)
Vegetable Dish	Onion and zucchini
	Salad—romaine lettuce with red onion, carrot, radish, cucumber
	Dressing: tahini, soy sauce, lemon juice
Pickle or Sour	Dill pickle (leftover salsa)
Salty Condiment	Gomashio

MONDAY — "INSPIRATION DAY - NEW GRAINS DAY"

BREAKFAST
Main Grain	Teff (2 pans - 1 with rice syrup and 1 without)
Second Grain	Oatmeal
Seeds/Nuts	Pumpkin seeds
Sweet Source	Rice syrup glaze for teff (one pan only)
Salt Source	Gomashio

LUNCH
Main Grain	Brown rice
Second Grain	Quinoa red lentil salad
Protein Source	(red lentils)
Fat Source	(sesame oil in soup, salad, and squash dish)
Soup/Bowl	Barley miso soup with bok choy, sauteed onion, carrot, wakame
Vegetable Dish	Yellow squash and onion, nitsuke style
	Light pressed cuke
Pickle or Sour	Dill pickle
Salty Condiment	Gomashio

SNACK   Pears

DINNER
Main Grain	Sushi with pickled ginger, walnuts, cucumber slices, carrots
Second Grain	(puffed cereal in dessert)
Protein Source	Scrambled tofu
Fat Source	(almonds, walnuts, peanut butter in dessert)
Soup/Bowl	Light miso onion soup with noodles
Vegetable Dish	Winter squash
	Blanched Chinese cabbage and carrot
Sea Vegetables	(nori in sushi)
Pickle or Sour	(pickled ginger in sushi)
Fruit/Dessert	Almond cereal munchie
Salty Condiment	Gomashio

TUESDAY — "EASY PREP" "VEGETABLE PICK-UP"

BREAKFAST
Main Grain	Oatmeal
Seeds/Nuts	Sunflower seeds
Sweet Source	Apple/raisin, pear pieces, cooked
Salt Source	Gomashio

LUNCH
Main Grain	Brown rice, plain
Second Grain	Rye crackers with peanut butter
Protein Source	(split pea soup, peanut butter)
Fat Source	(peanut butter, sesame oil in soup/cabbage dish)
Soup/Bowl	Split pea soup
Vegetable Dish	Sauteed cabbage with ume vinegar
	Boiled daikon with oily miso condiment
Sea Vegetables	Nori condiment
Pickle or Sour	Light pressed cuke pickles
Salty Condiment	(nori condiment, oily miso condiment)
	Gomashio

SNACK   Watermelon

DINNER
Main Grain	Brown rice
Second Grain	Spaghetti
Protein Source	(white beans)
Fat Source	(oil in sauce and sea palm)
Soup/Bowl	Minestrone soup with white beans
Vegetable Dish	Blanched broccoli
	Chunky sauce for spaghetti
Sea Vegetables	Sea palm
Pickle or Sour	Daikon pickle
Salty Condiment	Gomashio

WEDNESDAY — "NEW ENERGY INPUT REFRESH DAY" "CHAPATI CLASS"

BREAKFAST
Main Grain	Millet/quinoa
Second Grain	Oatmeal
Seeds/Nuts	Pumpkin seeds
Sweet Source	Prunes/raisins/orange pieces
Salt Source	Gomashio
	Roasted dulse

LUNCH
Main Grain	Brown rice
Second Grain	Tabouli on lettuce leaves
Protein Source	Fried tempeh served with sauerkraut
Fat Source	(fried tempeh)
Soup/Bowl	Kombu clear broth served with lemon garnish
Vegetable Dish	Corn on the cob
	Onion miso
	Blanched snow peas
Sea Vegetables	Kombu condiment
Pickle or Sour	(sauerkraut)
Salty Condiment	Gomashio

SNACK   Fruit platter—strawberry, peach

DINNER
Main Grain	Brown rice
Second Grain	Chapati from bread class
Protein Source	Humus
Fat Source	(tahini in humus)
Soup/Bowl	Light vegetable soup (onion, celery, corn, cabbage, daikon, barley miso)
Vegetable Dish	Green beans
Sea Vegetables	(kombu in beans)
Pickle or Sour	Cucumber relish (cukes, scallion, parsley, ginger juice, soy sauce, toasted sesame oil, lemon juice), served on lettuce leaf
Fruit/Dessert	Couscous cake with strawberry topping
Salty Condiment	Gomashio

THURSDAY — "CAMP WIND DOWN"

BREAKFAST
Main Grain	Oatmeal
Second Grain	Chapati or rice cakes with apple butter
Seeds/Nuts	Sunflower seeds
Sweet Source	Raisins
Salt Source	Gomashio

LUNCH
Main Grain	Brown rice
Second Grain	Pasta dish with sauteed onion, yellow squash, and carrot
Soup/Bowl	Barley miso soup with onion, celery, wakame, daikon
Vegetable Dish	Blanched kale
	Specialty dressing of soy sauce, olive oil, and brown rice vinegar
	(in noodle dish and soup)
Sea Vegetables	(wakame in soup)
Pickle or Sour	Sauerkraut
Salty Condiment	Gomashio

SNACK   Apples

DINNER
Main Grain	Long grain brown rice with wild rice
Protein Source	Azuki bean with winter squash
Fat Source	(oil in hijiki, salad dressing, nuts in cake)
Soup/Bowl	Corn chowder
Vegetable Dish	Salad: lettuce, radish, jicama, carrot, cucumber; dressing: ume, olive oil, lemon juice, herb
Sea Vegetables	Hijiki with sauteed onion, carrot, and sesame seed
Pickle or Sour	(ume and lemon in salad dressing)
Salty Condiment	Gomashio
Extra Dish	Popcorn for campfire

FRIDAY — "PARTY DAY" "VARIETY SHOW NIGHT"

BREAKFAST
Main Grain	Oatmeal
Second Grain	Polenta
Seeds/Nuts	Walnuts
Sweet Source	Strewed prunes
Salt Source	Gomashio
	Roasted dulse

LUNCH
Main Grain	Cornellia's 5-taste rice
Second Grain	Rye crackers with lentil pate
Protein Source	(lentil pate)
Fat Source	(tahini in pate, oil in soup and dressing)
Soup/Bowl	Barley miso soup with wakame, sauteed onion, cabbage, carrot
Vegetable Dish	Blanched baby bok choy
Sea Vegetables	(wakame in soup)
Pickle or Sour	Daikon pickle
Salty Condiment	Gomashio

SNACK   Apples and oranges

DINNER
Main Grain	Azuki bean rice cubbies
Second Grain	(millet with vegetable dish)
Protein Source	Seitan cutlets in sage gravy
Fat Source	(sage gravy with tahini and onion)
Soup/Bowl	(rice pudding)
Vegetable Dish	Cauliflower millet mashed potatoes
	Blanched green beans, carrots
Pickle or Sour	Sauerkraut
Fruit/Dessert	Rice pudding
Salty Condiment	Gomashio

SATURDAY — "LAST FULL DAY" "PACKING DAY"

BREAKFAST
Main Grain	Oatmeal
Second Grain	Bulghur or other grain
Seeds/Nuts	Sunflower or pumpkin seeds
Sweet Source	Raisins or other fruit
Salt Source	Gomashio

LUNCH
Main Grain	Brown rice
Second Grain	(couscous in vegetable dish)
Fat Source	(oil in soup)
	Almonds
	Bechamel sauce
Soup/Bowl	Barley miso soup with wakame, sauteed onion, red lentils, and other veggies
Vegetable Dish	Couscous
	Blanched cabbage or other vegetables
Sea Vegetables	(wakame in soup)
Pickle or Sour	Daikon pickle
Salty Condiment	Gomashio

SNACK   Apples or oranges

DINNER
Main Grain	Brown rice
Second Grain	Ohagi with sunflower seeds or walnuts
Protein Source	(black bean soup with seitan)
Fat Source	(oil in soup, sunflower seeds)
Soup/Bowl	Black bean soup with seitan
Vegetable Dish	Mixed Salad
Pickle or Sour	Daikon pickle or cucumber relish
Salty Condiment	Gomashio

SUNDAY — "HAPPY TRAILS DAY"

BREAKFAST
Main Grain	Oatmeal
Second Grain	Millet or other grain
Seeds/Nuts	Sunflower or pumpkin seeds
Sweet Source	Fruit
Salt Source	Gomashio

TRAVEL FOOD
Main Grain	Brown rice balls with nori and umeboshi
Second Grain	Trail mix
Protein Source	(nuts in trail mix)
Fat Source	(nuts in trail mix)
Vegetable Dish	Raw carrots and cucumbers and celery
Sea Vegetables	(nori on rice balls)
Pickle or Sour	(umeboshi in rice balls)
Fruit/Dessert	Apple and/or orange

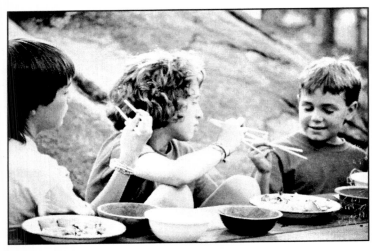

Learning Chopsticks at French Meadows Camp

Recipe Index

Almond delight cookies 80
Almonds, candied 95
Amaranth, steamed 119
Applesauce pudding 111
Arame and carrot 25
Arepas 98
Avocado sauerkraut toast, quick hors
    d'oeuvre 70
Avocado-olive spread 73
Azuki beans with winter squash 40

Bean soups 32
Beet, grated, with greens and orange 85
Black bean salsa 86
Black bean soup 34
Braised tempeh with green herb coulis 96
Bread, wayfarer's 120
Broccoli, blanched 23
Broth for soba 34
Buckwheat salad 18
Burdock ribs 77

Cabbage and onions 25
Cake, twelve-layer French Meadows 121
Candied almonds 95
Cantaloupe Pudding 68
Carrot daikon condiment 112
Carrot lime soup 85
Carrot salad, grated, with sweet rice
    vinegar 104
Carrot tofu aspic 67
Cauliflower and millet "mashed pota-
    toes" 27

Cauliflower curry coconut soup 90
Cereal, morning 103
Chickpea stew 63
Citrus-flax oil vinaigrette 95
Clear Soup, kombu 35
Cole slaw, quick-and-easy tangy 72
Compote 1, 12
Compote 2, 12
Compote 3, 13
Condiments 44
Congee recipe, basic 89
Corn chowder 31
Corn chowder, red lentil 64
Corn fritters 116
Corn on the cob 22
Couscous, fresh herb 106
Couscous, fried 116
Crackers 79
Crepes, sarrasin 120
Crookneck squash and onions 24
Cucumber relish 48
Cucumber salsa 48
Cucumbers, stuffed 113
Cucumber salad, wakame orange 47

Daikon condiment, carrot 112
Daikon with sweet miso sauce 115
Dipping sauce for pot stickers 87
Dressings 45
Dulse, roasted 12

Eggplant appetizer 74
European fried rice 112

Fermented veggies 78
Five-taste rice, 15
Flax sunflower basil umeboshi gomashio 108
Fresh green salsa 101
Fresh herb couscous 106
Fricassee, tempeh, mushroom, and celery 107

Gomashio, flax sunflower basil umeboshi 108
Green beans and carrots, blanched 24
Green herb coulis 96
Green salad, organic field, with candied almonds and sweet mustard-garlic vinaigrette 95
Greens, season's, and red radishes with citrus-flax oil vinaigrette 95
Greens with grated beet and orange 85

Halvah, macro 71
Hiziki side dish 83
Hummus, white bean, Italian, 84

Italian white bean hummus 84

Kabocha salad, steamed 69
Kale, radish greens, or baby bok choy, blanched 23
Kombu and shiitake condiment 45
Kombu clear soup, with or without shiitake mushroom 35
Kuzu Compote 71

Lemon Tahini Crush Cookies 92
Lentil paté 39

Marinade, basic 108
Millet 11
Millet "mashed potatoes," cauliflower 27
Minestrone soup 32
Minestrone soup, Packy's 78
Miso soup 30
Miso soup, hearty winter 30
Mixed media summer salad 104

Mochi pear melt, stovetop 68
Mochi, tempeh reuben 89
Mushroom, tempeh, and celery fricassee 107
Mustard-garlic vinaigrette, sweet 95

Nappa cabbage quinoa rolls with sesame sauce 88
Noodle and vegetable dish 26
Nori condiment 44

Oatmeal 10
Oily miso 44
Olive oil and umeboshi vinegar dressing 46
Onion miso 26
Onion soup, creamy 31

Parsnip delight 70
Pasta sauce, chunky 27
Pea soup 33
Peach compote, fresh 93
Peanut-apple-miso spread 75
Pickles, quick summer 71
Pilaf, three grain 108
Pinto beans and onions 86
Pot stickers 86
Prunes, stewed 12
Pumpkin seeds 10

Quick hors d'oeuvre: avocado sauerkraut toast 70
Quick summer pickles 71
Quinoa, cumin-scented, with shiitake mushroom sauce 93
Quinoa, Nappa cabbage, rolls with sesame sauce 88
Quinoa red lentil salad 17

Red lentil corn chowder 64
Red lentil salad, quinoa 17
Reuben, tempeh mochi 89
Rice, 5-taste 15
Rice cream 103
Rice croquettes 83

Rice, European fried 112
Rice salad, brown 17
Rice syrup sauce 13

Sage gravy 38
Salad, boiled 24
Salad, main course 119
Salad, mixed media summer 104
Salad, watercress 113
Salsa, black bean 86
Salsa, cucumber 48
Salsa verde cruda (fresh green salsa) 101
Sarrasin crepes 120
Seitan 36
Seitan cutlets 37
Seitan, fried 37
Sesame sauce 88
Shiitake condiment, kombu 45
Shiitake mushroom sauce 93
Side dishes 47
Snow peas, blanched 23
Soba summer salad 66
Spread, peanut-apple-miso 75
Strawberry couscous cake 110
Sunflower basil umeboshi gomashio, flax 108
Sunflower seeds 10
Sweet miso sauce 115
Sweet mustard-garlic vinaigrette 95

Tabouli salad 19
Tahini lemon ume salad dressing 46
Tamale filling 99
Tamales 99
Teff 11

Tempeh, braised with herb coulis 96
Tempeh mochi reuben 89
Tempeh, mushroom, and celery fricas-see 107
Three sister soup 118
Tofu 38
Tofu aspic, carrot 67
Tofu-pickle spread 74
Tofu, fried 39

Udon salad, spicy 91
Ume dill salad dressing 45
Umeboshi gomashio, flax sunflower basil 108
Umeboshi vinegar dressing, olive oil 46

Vegetable soups 31
Vegetables, grilled 107
Vegetables, mixed 24
Vegetables, solo 21
Vegetables, stir-fried 82
Vegetables, winter root, oven-roasted 106
Veggies, fermented, 78
Vinaigrette, citrus-flax oil 95
Vinaigrette, sweet mustard-garlic 95

Wakame cucumber salad 105
Wakame orange cucumber salad 47
Watercress salad 113
White bean hummus, Italian 84
White bean spread 73
White beans vinaigrette 75
Winter root vegetables, oven-roasted 106
Winter squash 22
Winter squash, with azuki beans 40